Blood Pressure Diet for Beginners

A Smart and Healthy Cookbook with Delicious Recipes in Order to reduce your Blood Pressure, Learn How reducing Blood Pressure is the best Antiviral, Prevent all Heart Diseases and Maintain Weight Loss Eating

By

Paul Heller and K. Diamond

© Copyright 2020 by Paul Heller and K.Diamond - All rights reserved.

This document is geared towards providing exact and reliable information in regards to the topic and issue covered. The publication is sold with the idea that the publisher is not required to render accounting, officially permitted or otherwise qualified services. If advice is necessary, legal or professional, a practiced individual in the profession should be ordered.

- From a Declaration of Principles which was accepted and approved equally by a Committee of the American Bar Association and a Committee of Publishers and Associations.

In no way is it legal to reproduce, duplicate, or transmit any part of this document in either electronic means or in printed format. Recording of this publication is strictly prohibited, and any storage of this document is not allowed unless with written permission from the publisher. All rights reserved.

The information provided herein is stated to be truthful and consistent, in that any liability, in terms of inattention or otherwise, by any usage or abuse of any policies, processes, or directions contained within is the solitary and utter responsibility of the recipient reader. Under no circumstances will any legal responsibility or blame be held against the publisher for any reparation, damages, or monetary loss due to the information herein, either directly or indirectly.

Respective authors own all copyrights not held by the publisher.

The information herein is offered for informational purposes solely and is universal as so. The presentation of the information is without a contract or any type of guarantee assurance.

The trademarks that are used are without any consent, and the publication of the trademark is without permission or backing by the trademark owner. All trademarks and brands within this book are for clarifying purposes only and are owned by the owners themselves, not affiliated with this document.

Table Of Contents

INTRODUCTION 7

CHAPTER 1: UNDERSTANDING BLOOD PRESSURE 10

1.1 Types of Blood Pressure 10

1.2 High Blood Pressure Measurement 12

1.3 Causes of High Blood Pressure 16

1.4 Bringing Down High Blood Pressure 21

1.5 High Blood Pressure the Number One Killer 22

1.6 How Often Should You Be Checked? 23

1.7 Elevated Blood Pressure Associated Diseases 24

1.8 Lack of Awareness Is Dangerous 25

1.9 Is This an Issue That Is Increasing or Decreasing? 26

CHAPTER 2: HIGH BLOOD PRESSURE PROBLEMS 28

2.1 Heart Issues 29

2.2 Diabetes 33

2.3 Kidney Problems 33

2.4 Increased Cholesterol Levels 35

2.5 Problems Requiring Beta or Alpha-Blockers 36

2.6 Blood-Thinning Drugs 38

2.7 Racial Variations 39

2.8 Pain–Particularly Joint Pain and Arthritis 39

2.9 Psychological Problems 42

CHAPTER 3: MEDICATION AND BLOOD PRESSURE ... 44

3.1 High Blood Pressure Medications and Their Roles 44

3.2 Other Medicines Often Used to Treat High Blood Pressure 45

3.3 Resistant Hypertension: 47

3.4 Vitamin Supplement Recommendations 48

3.5 Effectiveness of Weight Management While Elevating Blood Pressure Problems 52

CHAPTER 4: SUPPLEMENT AND EXERCISE 57

4.1 One Move That Helps Lower Your Blood Pressure without Medication 57

4.2 Can Low-Intensity Exercise Like Walking Reduce Your Blood Pressure? 58

4.3 How Much Exercise Do You Need to Keep Your Blood Pressure Under Control? 58

4.4 What Will Make It Easier to Stick to A Daily Exercise? 59

4.5 The 6 Best Exercises to Reduce High Blood Pressure 60

4.6 Supplements to Lower Blood Pressurevist 62

CHAPTER 5: DEALING WITH BLOOD PRESSURE IN DAILY LIFE 68

5.1 Which Diet Is Best? 68

5.2 Preventive Snacking 69

5.3 Stop Stress Eating 70

5.4 Learning Portion Control 72

5.5 Lose Excess Pounds and Watch Your Waistline. 74

5.6 Relieve Stress. 74

5.7 Other Blood Pressure Management Tips 75

CHAPTER 6: HEALTHY RECIPES TO CONTROL BLOOD PRESSURE AND LOSE WEIGHT 79

6.1 Some Foods That Help Lower Blood Pressure 79

6.2 Appetizers 83

6.3 Beverages 95

6.4 Breads 103

6.5 Salads 112

6.6 Soups 122

6.7 Vegetables or Side Dishes 130

6.8 Entrees 142

6.9 Marinades, Seasonings, and Rubs 156

6.10 Desserts 160

CONCLUSION 174

REFERENCES 175

Introduction

Whereas you picked this book out of basic curiosity or desire, this cookbook is built to make life on a low-sodium diet easy and enjoyable. To those that are new to the diet, dash is an acronym to dietary approaches to stop hypertension. This cookbook is a healthy, balanced diet low in sodium and high in fruits, vegetables, whole grains, and low-fat dairy products. Meats, candy, and nuts are all allowed, but the added sugars and fats should be consumed in moderation.

A low-sodium diet is frequently recommended for people with severe medical conditions. It is shown to help the body recover by reducing blood pressure, decreasing cholesterol, and encouraging heart safety and wellbeing in general. Like with other smart eating plans, it has the added benefit of encouraging safe weight loss and weight maintenance and can even help avoid obesity, osteoporosis, and diabetes. In short, the blood pressure diet cookbook for beginners can help millions of people live longer, safer lives.

Yet to benefit from this, you must commit! By reality, because of their impracticability, many fall short of dietary objectives. Modern lives are always busy, and, as a result, eating healthy sometimes takes a back seat before a health crisis erupts. Blood pressure diet cookbook for beginners has published with this in mind. With simple, inexpensive, and delicious recipes — all with 30 minutes or less of cooking time — there is no reason not to prioritize yourself and your health.

In blood pressure diet cookbook for beginners, you'll enjoy many of the same things you've always eaten: fresh fruits and vegetables, low-fat dairy products, whole grains, beans, meats, and desserts.

You're not going to feel cheated! But you're going to need to adapt. Salt-free living isn't comfortable, but it's worth it because it's worth it! Freeing yourself from the stigma of poor health is a task that needs to be taken to heart (pun intended).

The first step in beginning the diet is simple: stop using salt. From there, you'll need to store a low-sodium pantry, searching for items specifically designed for a salt-free, low-sodium audience. It helps to buy a small food book, so you are comfortable with the sodium content of most popular foods. You may want to hold it in your wallet or pocket and use it when shopping or dining out.

The good news is that you can either buy or make anything you need to survive on a regular dash diet. And as low-sodium foods become more popular, companies are gradually responding to demand by widening product lines, making salt-free cooking even simpler and more convenient.

You are using the recipes and details in this book to ignite your imagination. Wherever you stay, search, and browse for items that meet low sodium requirements (140 mg or less per serving). Engage with the world around you, visiting local farms and farmers' markets, to buy the freshest and cheapest items, ideally organic wherever possible. New recipes will naturally evolve out of every season, and by adding the freshest ingredients, you'll give your body the best you can. Instead of diet alone, explore every path at your fingertips for a healthy lifestyle. Join a gym, take a fitness class, or even go outside and take a walk, if possible, every day.

I look forward to spending your time taking care of yourself.

A low-sodium diet is something you need to stick to seriously. You can't give up and hope to make inroads. It may be challenging, but don't give it up.

The body is going to thank you! For the days when you feel like you're just floating in the cold, remember: you're in the sea! Someone above you on the bleachers will see your improvement, even though you can't. You may be struggling with exhaustion, but with everyday practice, you are building stamina, and eventually, performance.

Chapter 1: Understanding Blood Pressure

Blood pressure is the pressure exerted on the walls of the blood vessel as blood travels into the arteries. Blood vessels serve as blood pipes and carry it to body tissues and organs from the pumping heart. Blood is pumped out of the heart each time the heartbeats, which causes the pressure to increase. Between pulses, the heart refills with blood while the heart is at rest, and the pressure decreases in the arteries.

Problems occur when the heart fills up again, but the pressure in the arteries persists or even increases at the same point. This induces excess strain in the arteries and strains the walls of the arteries. The discomfort is known as hypertension. Blood pressure depends on two factors: cardiac production, or blood volume pumped out of the heart, and peripheral blood vessel resistance to blood flow through the circulatory system.

Find the circulatory system to be a garden hose. The water pressure in a garden hose may be increased by opening the faucet to allow a larger volume of water or by tightening the nozzle to restrict the spray, which reduces the resistance to water flow. The circulatory system functions likewise. The overall amount of blood that the heart pumps out is determined by the total volume of fluid in the blood vessels, as well as the heart pumping rate and effectiveness. The scale of the tiny arteries influences the system strain. These small arteries have the muscle fibers in their walls, which can cause them to constrict or dilate, controlling blood flow in the "pipe network." if you cut off part, what kinds of high bp are there?

1.1 Types of Blood Pressure

There are and indeed are more than we know.

BLOOD PRESSURE CATEGORY	SYSTOLIC mm Hg (upper number)		DIASTOLIC mm Hg (lower number)
NORMAL	LESS THAN 120	and	LESS THAN 80
ELEVATED	120 – 129	and	LESS THAN 80
HIGH BLOOD PRESSURE (HYPERTENSION) STAGE 1	130 – 139	or	80 – 89
HIGH BLOOD PRESSURE (HYPERTENSION) STAGE 2	140 OR HIGHER	or	90 OR HIGHER
HYPERTENSIVE CRISIS (consult your doctor immediately)	HIGHER THAN 180	and/or	HIGHER THAN 120

High bp was historically divided into two major groups:

• Rare cases with known causes (secondary hypertension, that is, high bp due to other conditions) and

• Standard instances in which there is no known cause (essential hypertension). Necessary' didn't mean high bp was required because it was' critical': you've got it, and you've had it, for reasons you've had it unclear.

The word ' primary hypertension' or' primary high bp' is now starting to give way to common sense terminology.

Secondary elevated bp is often caused by various kinds of kidney failure or usually by aorta malformations ("coarctation"), overproduction of certain bp-rearing hormones by hypophysis tumors, adrenal glands, or kidney tumors, or my brain or brain injury stress conditions. These' classical' indirect causes make up less than 1% of all cases of elevated bp diagnosed. That holds valid even if we remove elevated bp caused by oral contraceptive pills.

Because' significant' high bp is an unexplained cause by itself, the category eventually is more surreal, as there are more overlapping triggers. We now know a variety of leading reasons which, if treated in an early stage, could lead to a drop in bp, but these were not yet listed as' secondary hypertension.' types include overweight and alcohol intake for young people, especially those who have a family history of high bp and who are genetically susceptible to these causes. As more specific objectives are discovered, even primary hypertension must eventually be classified as a separate category.

1.2 High Blood Pressure Measurement

The blood pressure determined by the application of mercury consists of two artery forces: systolic and diastolic. The top number is the systolic pressure created when the heart contracts. The second number refers to diastolic pressure produced by calming the heart between the beats. The average calculation of blood pressure is the peak degree in the lower (systolic/diastolic). A person has an average blood pressure of no more than 120/80 mmHg. Blood pressure is considered normal between 120/80 mmHg and130/8 five mmHg, with values of 130/85 mmHg and 139/89 mmHg being considered high. High and extremely elevated blood pressure is referred to as the systolic blood pressure of 180 mmHg or above and the diastolic blood pressure of 120 mmHg or more.

High blood pressure is defined by the American heart association and the national heart, lung, and blood institute (NHLBI) as one or two facts: dystopian forces of 140 mm or higher mercury and a diastolic pressure of 90 mm or more mercury.

Take Drugs to Reduce Blood Pressure

Individual blood pressure can differ in particular whether patients are anxious or excited during a visit to a doctor. The blood pressure level in adults is based on the average of 2 or more accurately calculated levels of sitting blood pressure for one of 2 or more office visits. Studies say ambulatory monitoring blood pressure, which provides an average 24-hour blood pressure level, may provide a better clinical high blood pressure indicator.

Prehypertension or-high blood pressure was known as American, where the blood pressure is higher than average but not hypertension. The 7th joint national committee report (jnc 7) introduced a revised concept of below 140/90 mmHg blood pressure levels. Pre-high blood pressure measurements with the systolic pressure between 120 mmHg and 139 mmHg or with the diastolic pressure between 80 mm and 89 mmHg are considered. High blood pressure levels higher than or equal to 140/90 mmHg are considered.

Over the years, the concept of elevated blood pressure has shifted.

We now realize that people with reduced blood pressure have significantly improved cardiovascular function in the long run.

If the systemic and diastolic pressure drops into different levels, a person with elevated blood pressure or low blood pressure is identified by a higher set of values. Increased diastolic blood pressure was historically considered as a risk factor more severe than systolic changes, but chronically elevated blood pressure now tends to be a higher risk.

The doctors address the aggressiveness and perceived importance that people who do not sustain such control on their use to lower stresses within the usual range.

Treatment of elevated blood pressure is essential to prevent skyrocketing to alarming rates that can lead to strokes, heart problems, and aortic aneurysms.

Such results indicate that people with high pressure will use reduced sugar, low sodium, and mild carbohydrate diets.

¨consult with her psychiatrist on elevated blood pressure, high cholesterol, and diabetic drugs.

Hold a Diabetes Care Class

Walk a few blocks and walk up to one mile each day.

Reduce stress with yoga or calming strategies and take less demanding work options into account.

Eat fish which is high in omega-3 fatty acids than red meat.

Replace standard salad dressings for sweet, low-sodium, or fat-free dressings.

Drink 64 ounces a day of beer.

Create her favorite list of nutritious foods.

Learn to buy and consume low glycemic indices meals for improved blood sugar control.

Increase the average fruit and vegetable consumption.

Reduce the fruit juice intake to 4 ounces a day and then eat whole grains.

Reduce the salt intake and search for low-sodium shopping items.

Several acute, life-threatening complications can be caused by seven studies from the joint national committee for the prevention, diagnosis, assessment, and care of high-blood pressure (the jnc 7 report). They are called high blood pressure emergencies.

It can include elevated blood pressure encephalopathy, vomiting, or inflammation in the eye and acute insufficiency in the kidney. Low blood pressure incidents may be confusing — severe blood pressure accidents, malignant high blood pressure, emergency for elevated blood pressure, and rapid high blood pressure are all common. The treatment of an emergency elevated blood pressure not only depends on the actual blood pressure level but also the previous average blood pressure level of a patient. Such accidents tend to be the most frequent in people who are not diagnosed or who have not taken a prescription drug system.

High blood pressure can, however, also occur in people who take medicines as instructed. In the case of elevated blood pressure crises, one or more drugs will gradually reduce blood pressure.

The ability to not reduce blood pressure too quickly is significant because a sudden decrease in blood pressure will lead to heart, brain, or kidney injury.

Measuring the Blood Pressure at Home

Blood pressure levels will differ from tests obtained in the office and hospital environment of the typical doctor. However, home readings can be useful in determining signs indicative of elevated blood pressure as such signs are not always apparent within the few minutes of a regular physician's visit to the hospital. Household screening will also be a helpful way of controlling elevated blood pressure.

Those who test blood pressure at home have a benefit because they rely on monitoring the disease. Real blood pressure can be measured even more precisely by a sequence of home readings than by one or two "casual" blood pressure (bp) tests at the workplace.

Home readings can be a valuable complement to knowledge gathered in the office of the physician, especially when the two are widely disparate. Long-term tests have found that those with significantly lower bp levels at home experience less significant coronary problems than those who have higher levels at home and in the workplace. The same methods can be used in doctor's offices when calculating blood pressure at home. Then sit comfortably for two to five minutes, then make sure the blood pressure cuff's "bladder" occupies 80% of the arm's circumference. Make this sure that you are sitting comfortably and rest your neck parallel to the core and palm up in the sleeve.

Individuals with elevated blood pressure should maintain an accurate list of levels of blood pressure and the day and date they will be expected to discuss with their doctor for the next visit. Each system that is used at home will satisfy aggressive medical instrument advancement requirements. If home measurements are taken, otherwise, a normal sphygmomanometer will be used to calibrate the home measuring instrument.

Such blood pressure monitoring devices are advised at home: a&d medical life source those dealing with extremely high blood pressure can benefit from daily blood pressure checks as a safe approach to control high blood pressure. You're inspired by the effects of improvements in exercise and diet. It will also help you determine how well the drug controls the blood pressure, whether you are taking medication.

1.3 Causes of High Blood Pressure

In some cases, it is impossible to determine the precise cause of the elevated blood pressure. This "unspecified-cause" blood pressure is known as high blood pressure necessary, or high blood pressure main.

That can sound a little confounding before you realize it is necessarily indicative of something. Individuals have their own genetic and biochemical structure. Inherent and unchangeable features include ÿ heredity: whether either or more of their parents have elevated blood pressure, people are at higher risk.

Men are at a marginally higher risk than women, but women's elevated blood pressure is often undiagnosed and untreated.

Age: the risk of elevated blood pressure increases with age.

Race: African Americans are at higher risk.

Let's look in more depth at the effects of class, age, and race.

Sex

If you're xx (female), or if you're xy (male), are you more likely to have high blood pressure?

This is a question many patients are wondering, and the picture is very mixed. Many of the men and women are considered to have the same chances with elevated blood pressure. Nonetheless, people could be more likely to experience hypertension before age 55.

Age

The need to control elevated blood pressure isn't minimized by becoming older.

On the opposite, as people age, there are all the same health problems, but other associated factors are rising, such as the possibility of high blood pressure. When people grow older, their muscles grow stiffer, and blood pressure continues to rise naturally.

There are many benefits of reducing elevated systolic blood pressure in adults, and scientific trials indicate considerable advantages in controlling high blood pressure in later life years.

17

Healthy aging is a beautiful cycle, and new findings show a reduction in elevated blood pressure and medical diseases such as heart disease or stroke among seniors who follow a healthy lifestyle.

Projections by the census bureau said that by the year 2050, the number of Americans over 65 would well reach 100 million. Despite these numbers, efforts to help older Americans control elevated blood pressure and associated conditions need to be redoubled.

Race

The high blood pressure rate in African Americans ranks among the worst in the country. This means more African Americans have high blood pressure than the other minority groups. In comparison, African Americans are reporting a comparatively lower incidence of diagnosis and treatment with elevated blood pressure.

African Americans experience high blood pressure early in life compared to the Caucasians, and average blood pressure in African Americans is significantly higher. The average incidence of elevated blood pressure in adult African Americans is considerably higher than in Caucasians (28.1 percent vs. 23.2 percent). But high blood pressure among young adult African Americans, particularly young women, is far more common. High blood pressure, for example, happens in 8.5 percent of white women and 22.9 percent of African American women in the 35 to 44 age group. High blood pressure affects one-third of all African American women.

Like in other races, African Americans often do not seek care after long stretches of blood pressure have been raised, and significant organ failure is present.

The African American population has a much higher prevalence of illness and mortality associated with elevated blood pressure, including end-stage kidney disease.

African Americans have an 80 percent higher mortality rate for strokes, a 50 percent higher mortality rate for heart failure, and a more than 300 percent prevalence for elevated blood pressure-related end-stage renal failure than seen in the general population.

African Americans seeking appropriate care may undergo comparable average decreases in blood pressure relative to Caucasians and can have a lower rate of cardiovascular disease.

While African Americans tend to be suffering the most with this disease, it also affects other ethnicities significantly. Heart diseases are the foremost cause of death in all races, and the correlation between elevated blood pressure and heart disease is significant.

Throughout the United States, the prevalence of blood pressure regulation for Hispanics is lower than in the Caucasians and African Americans. Asian-American / Pacific Islander women have significantly lower screening rates for blood pressure than other minority groups, while elevated blood pressure is a big concern for these groups. Both Native Americans and Alaskan natives, this is the reverse. In a new study conducted by the centers for disease control, survey respondents addressed the question, "did a nurse, doctor, or other health care provider ever tell you that you have elevated blood pressure? "The study showed that Native Americans / Alaska residents had a higher incidence of elevated blood pressure than the national average. Both racial groups definitely should pay careful attention to blood pressure.

When we speak about ethnicity-related high blood pressure, we apply to critical high blood pressure, as described earlier.

A better term to characterize critical high blood pressure is primary high blood pressure, which, apart from genetic causes, means that there is no clear medical explanation to justify the condition of a patient. We may differentiate between primary hypertension and secondary blood pressure.

Think about it this way: a ripple effect will cause complications with elevated blood pressure when something goes wrong with one area of the body. In secondary high blood pressure, the high blood pressure condition stems from or is due to another disorder, such as diabetes mellitus, other forms of cancers, and kidney failure. In fact, according to the American heart association, 5 to 10 percent of elevated blood pressure cases are caused by an underlying disorder. Secondary blood pressure begins to pop up unexpectedly. But the positive news is that care proper will also regulate or reverse both the underlying disease and elevated blood pressure. While elevated blood pressure may not necessarily be an immediate cause, controlling high blood pressure decreases the risk of severe risks like heart disease, stroke, and kidney failure.

Another piece of the puzzle is that several risk factors can exacerbate or cause hypertension. There are decisions about lifestyle and environmental influences.

Alcohol: blood pressure rises with heavy drinking.

Weight: the higher the overweight, the greater the risk of having high blood pressure.

Smoking: nicotine shrinks tiny blood vessels, increasing blood pressure.

Contraceptive and hormone use: in people who are on the pill who use contraceptive patches who NuvaRing, blood pressure rises, mainly when people often consume alcohol and smoke cigarettes.

Sodium consumption: certain people with their diet or drink are susceptible to sodium content. The high blood hazards

1.4 Bringing Down High Blood Pressure

Blood pressure increases when people who are prone to salts ingest some sort of spice. For African Americans, that is especially so. For 45 to 50 percent of all individuals with elevated blood pressure, salt exposure is present.

Sedentary lifestyle: lack of physical activity means the heart is less powerful, and the sound and strength of the blood vessels is lower.

Extra blood flow and weight gain during pregnancy can increase blood pressure in women, particularly women with a family history of higher blood pressure, even though blood pressure was regularly normal before pregnancy.

Repressed frustration and unmanaged tension: some studies suggest that individuals who do not communicate their rage/emotions or who have extreme stress have a higher chance of elevated blood pressure and heart attacks.

Medicines are used for other disorders (e.g., decongestants) such as over-counter and asthma drug antihistamines.

The misuse of street drugs will lead to a dramatic increase in blood pressure from both drug intoxication and additives used to decrease the value of pure narcotics. There have been cases of fatal strokes of young cocaine users.

Less alarming are the causes of elevated blood pressure than long-term consequences. If left untreated, chronically high blood pressure can result in strokes, heart attacks, cardiac disease, aneurysm of the arteries, and kidney failure. And mild blood pressure elevations result in reduced life expectancy.

Newer Drugs for Blood Pressure Lowered the Risk of This Side Effect.

At some point in his adult life, virtually every man struggles to attain an erection tight enough for intercourse. More than 35 million American men have chronic issues of construction being obtained and sustained. Numerous erectile dysfunction medications had an economic impact due to the occurrence of this disease. Such medications benefit about 80 percent of people by increasing blood supply to the penis. Still, these miracle drugs do not support men with elevated blood pressure, diabetes, coronary disease, and other degenerative disorders that harm the nerves in the penis. Difficulty having or holding an erection is the result of decreased blood flow to the penis, which sometimes starts with blood supplying narrowed or blocked arteries to it. The arteries in the penis are small. Hence, a readily identified issue is erectile dysfunction, this can be the first sign or symptom of elevated blood pressure so cardiovascular disease. Impotence may also be an early warning indication that arteries are already being lined by plaque in some regions of the body that can raise the risk of heart disease and stroke.

1.5 High Blood Pressure the Number One Killer

High blood pressure is a significant public health crisis that can only escalate as the population ages. High blood pressure in the United States affects about one in four people. Nearly half of Americans age 55 and over have elevated blood pressure, so you are at higher risk if you're male, so over 35. In the United States, the average risk of having elevated blood pressure reaches a whopping 90 percent. At extreme high pressure, which is characterized as 50 percent or more above normal mean arterial pressure, a person may expect to live for no longer than a few years unless the condition is adequately treated.

Arteries transport oxygen-carrying blood to the heart muscle, and if the heart is unable to provide enough oxygen, there might be chest pain, commonly known as angina. Blocking the blood supply results in a heart attack.

1.6 How Often Should You Be Checked?

The 29-year-old heart attack is more severe than most people believe. Heart disease affects more people than any other death — 1.5 million deaths a year. Many people do not know that heart disease takes as many lives as the next five leading causes of death combined: stroke, untreated lower respiratory disorders, injuries, diabetes mellitus, and influenza/pneumonia. The truth is far from bleak. For example, a drop in diastolic blood pressure by just 5 to 6 mmHg decreases the risk of heart failure by 20 percent.

A lot of people avoid visiting the hospital. There is an excellent risk of sickness or the detection the adverse health problems. Therefore, people feel embarrassed because they have not accepted the instructions of a doctor for weight loss, drug intake, or smoking cessation. Health premiums and health care will also find it impossible to adjust the physicians. Nonetheless, don't be afraid to carry on looking for a doctor who knows you as a patient and can work for you positively. Depending on your medical needs, the doctor may also be a general medicine practitioner or internist or maybe a cardiology expert.

One crucial medical recommendation is how much you will get a blood pressure test or a checkup. Your doctor will use your patient profile to determine an appropriate time for monitoring your blood pressure.

Most physicians agree that for most patients with elevated blood pressure, semi-annual appointments are required to ensure the adequacy of blood pressure management, manage weight and other modifiable risk factors screening, and check and update medications. A semi-annual visit also calls for additional sessions to follow up on dietary changes and modifications to the prescription.

Medication is a vital aspect of a lot of people controlling elevated blood pressure. It is important to remember that in most cases, medicine would not be as effective in reducing high blood pressure if people don't make long-term lifestyle changes. The drug can adversely interfere with your environment, diet, and intake of other substances.

As Jason found, the first drug he took for his metabolism was not the right one. I will offer a more detailed description of blood pressure drugs in the report. When you make significant improvements in behavior, you may be able to will or remove the drug entirely. You will also reduce the chances of contracting diseases related to blood pressure.

1.7 Elevated Blood Pressure Associated Diseases

High blood pressure doesn't only cause heart failure. The most significant risk factor for stroke is changes in blood pressure. Very high blood pressure can lead to a crack in a compromised blood vessel, which then bleeds in the brain, which can lead to a stroke. If one of the shortened arteries is crossed by a blood clot that may also cause a stroke.

High blood pressure has also been related to an eye injury. High blood pressure can cause blood vessels to burst or leak in the eye.

Vision can get blurred or otherwise affected and can lead to blindness. Glaucoma was also related to hypertension.

When humans mature, arteries harden throughout the body, particularly those in the heart, brain, and kidneys. Such "stiffer" arteries are associated with elevated blood pressure. It, in turn, triggers more work for the heart and kidneys. When the organs function harder, they may get weakened, which also leads to the failure of the kidneys.

1.8 Lack of Awareness Is Dangerous

Because elevated blood pressure is closely linked with heart disease and other illnesses, education is vital. Nonetheless, according to the national health and nutrition examination survey, it is up to only over 70 percent of people with elevated blood pressure! Blood pressure management levels are reduced in conscious patients who are undergoing elevated blood pressure care. Ultimately, according to the study, the disorder is regulated by just 35 percent of people with high blood pressure.

High blood pressure remains a prevalent issue following many advancements and recent discoveries that would alleviate the problem, including the availability of more high blood pressure drugs than at any other point in history.

There are many suggested explanations for this, and it is not just one person that is responsible for the blame. Providers of health insurance, health-care programs, and consumers all play a part. Between health care providers, there is also a difference in the management of elevated blood pressure between the national recommendations and current clinical practice. Alas, many physicians are also not involved in helping their patients control blood pressure at optimal levels. To confuse the issue more, many doctors don't stick to elevated blood pressure care plans. About 45 percent of high blood pressure patients are reported to follow dietary changes or routinely and reliably take drugs.

Most doctors are taking medicine but do little to combat the underlying cause of elevated blood pressure.

Specific obstacles to hospital blood pressure management are lack of primary care coverage and lack of health insurance. But if people try to control their blood pressure, some lack the tools to help them do so effectively.

In selective populations, the devastating impact of not controlling elevated blood pressure is especially apparent. Since elevated blood pressure is more common in older women than in older people, a greater risk of mortality from high blood pressure results in older women. In older women, sixty percent of deaths related explicitly to untreated, elevated blood pressure occur. Similarly, among African Americans, the higher prevalence of elevated blood pressure results in a significantly higher rate of fatal stroke, coronary attack death, and renal dysfunction than in other ethnic groups.

Whether you have been hospitalized with elevated blood pressure lately, or have had the disease for years, you need to control your blood pressure to prevent life-threatening complications. When you've taken the time to read this book, you've already won a portion of the fight because you're in the right mood and ready to learn how to lower your blood pressure. You're inspired to better your health after hearing about the risks of high blood pressure.

Throughout the following pages, we will include tips and recommendations on nutritious, salt-free eating, weight loss, and exercising to help bring down your high blood pressure.

1.9 Is This an Issue That Is Increasing or Decreasing?

There is little indication that the general public has undergone a significant change in bp in the 70 or so years that statistics are available.

There is some evidence from the United States that it could have declined, and that this decline is attributed to the use of bp-decreasing medications over the past 30 years. Whatever definition of high bp is used (and that has changed a lot, as both meanings are arbitrary), the percentage of individuals with high bp is closely related to normal population strain.

Standardized and precise calculations of bp for large representative populations have been possible only since the 1950s in the UK, Scandinavia, and the USA, and more recently for other nations. There is some evidence from countries whose national diet has changed from very high to much lower sodium intakes, especially Japan, Portugal, and Belgium, that average bp has dropped in the general population, perhaps for this reason. Such sodium intake reductions reflect changes in food storage practices from salting, cooking, and pickling, to fresh food refrigeration and quick transport. As these developments have arisen in all economically developing countries, bp has undoubtedly declined everywhere relative to 19th-century average rates.

This opinion is reinforced by patterns in stroke-related mortality rates, which are considered to depend more on average bp than any other cause. Stroke rates have plummeted in every nation that gathers full and accurate statistics on deaths by medically approved purpose, perhaps since the 1920s, definitely since the 1950s.

Blood pressure and hypertension because you are costly rather than inadequate, are you more likely to have high bp?

No, it's precisely the reverse. Studies found higher average bps in the most impoverished communities. While these bp variations are not significant in different social groups, there are also variations in other heart disease risk factors.

Such disparities turn into changes in rates of stroke and heart attack among each group.

Chapter 2: High Blood Pressure Problems

Rarely is elevated blood pressure a particular disorder. Low bp happens most frequently in combination with other medical issues. Such disorders may alter the risk of stroke or heart attack (cardiovascular disease) of an individual or cause bp medications to be' tailored.'

Health attacks, asthma, and renal failure are all diseases associated with a higher risk of these complications, so if bp is still elevated, doctors will put you on target-level bp-lowering medications. Other factors discussed in this chapter are not correlated in themselves with elevated risk but have significant consequences in terms of choosing the best drug for you.

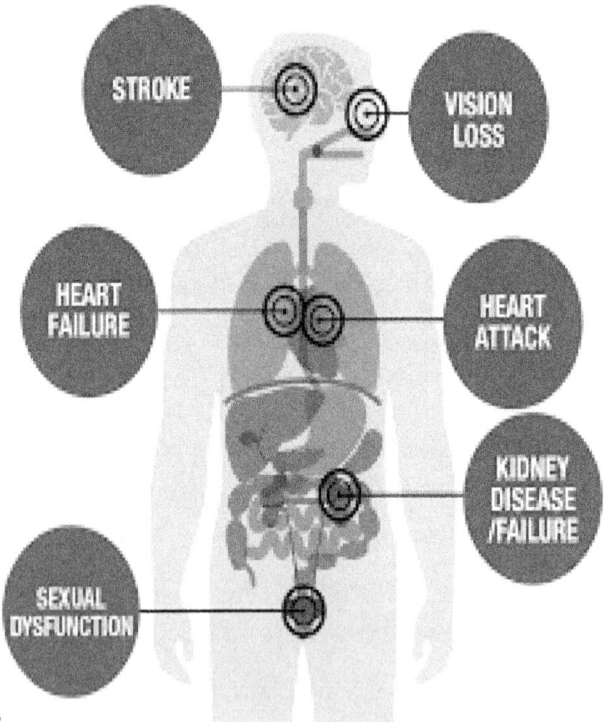

2.1 Heart Issues

I think I'm overweight and have trouble stopping smoking. You've spoken about risk factors that can raise my odds of having a heart attack or stroke. Where does all this apply to what medications to May my bp are chosen?

A risk assessment is essential to pick the best medications for you and specific circumstances. Comprehensive risk management helps to classify all significant risk factors that may need care as well as elevated bp. They will also determine the total benefit that every patient should obtain from different medication and non-drug treatments. There could be other risks for some individuals that take priority over handling elevated bp. For example, someone with wretched chronic obstructive airways disease and urinary incontinence has more urgent issues in terms of quality of life and alleviation of pain than the introduction of another set of medications, which may make treatment of their obstructive airways' disease and urinary incontinence easier.

Prioritizing care for patients like yourself with likely numerous cardiovascular risk factors and coexisting conditions is very difficult for both health providers and the patient. It is a time-consuming and challenging method to make choices on which risks take priority and whether care can be adapted to resolve these. Data on the different threats are widely visible in the media. You ought to weigh the potential advantages and disadvantages, the relationship of opioid therapy for high bp with any other problems you might have, and what your interest and expectations for life-long care maybe before deciding for specific treatments.

I was diagnosed with angina, and now I've got high bp to top it all. What medications would benefit me the most?

Individuals with angina or those who have suffered a heart attack ('myocardial infarction') are by definition at high risk of another attack. Beta-blockers have been found to have significant effects of both relieving angina symptoms and reducing the risk of death from heart attacks of individuals with a history of angina, particularly notably in those people who have had a previous heart attack. Despite this, beta-blockers are often used as the first elevated bp treatment. Calcium-channel antagonists may also give symptomatic angina relief. It has been shown that ace inhibitor drugs are highly effective in reducing mortality, mainly if you are at very high risk for cardiovascular disease. Calcium-channel antagonists are not used in individuals with a history of heart disease who also suffer from heart failure.

Just I had a heart attack, and now I have heart disease. Which are the most potent medications for my elevated bp, and what remedies do I avoid?

The ace inhibitors are the safest therapy in people with heart disease.

We have been found to decrease the risk of death regardless of the extent of heart disease.

Receptor blockers for angiotensin ii have also found to be particularly successful in people with heart disease. They are usually used as second-line medications in patients in whom ace inhibitor side effects are problematic or in which heart failure signs are not adequately alleviated. Beta-blockers are also ideal for heart disease and can be used in patients with heart failure for bp control with added benefits.

Alpha-adrenoceptor blocking medications and long-acting calcium channel blockers are related to deteriorating heart disease and increasing death risk.

I have an irregular heartbeat caused by what they call' atrial fibrillation,' which my doctor says. How exactly is that, and how does it affect my high bp management?

Atrial fibrillation means the rapid and uncoordinated activity of the heart muscle fibers, so that they form an inefficient, sweating mass rather than acting appropriately together to squeeze blood into the heart. If that occurs in the heart's central chambers, the' ventricles,' the heart fails, and you die until anyone can interrupt that cycle by providing an electrical shock to the core. Just the two upper and less essential chambers of the heart, the auricles, or atria cause atrial fibrillation.

Atrial fibrillation is prevalent, particularly among those over 70 years of age. Occasionally normal heart function can be recovered, either by medication or by a regulated electrical shock, often followed by a pacemaker implant to preserve regular service. It is uncommonly vital. The most significant problem is preventing the development of blood clots in the heart's atrial chambers using anticoagulants such as warfarin or aspirin.

Blood-thinning has been found to avoid dislodging of the clots in the atria, transfer to the brain, and cause a stroke. When you have atrial fibrillation, consider taking a sort of thinning blood medication to minimize the risk. Your risk of suffering a stroke will be determined by your age (your risk of stroke increases as you get older), whether or not you have suffered a stroke or a mini-stroke ('transient ischemic attack' or tia) in the past, whether you suffer from heart failure or whether you suffer from high blood pressure.

Most patients who have heart disease recover from atrial fibrillation, too.

Treatment with ace inhibitors, diuretics, and sometimes digoxin, to slow their heart rate and increase heart output for most people with heart failure, alleviates symptoms and improves their quality of life. They also take a type of blood-thinning drug to reduce their risk of stroke.

It is probably one of the significant causes of heart disease because you already have elevated bp. Paradoxically, when the heart falls, the bp will begin to decrease and raise when heat loss is regulated and cardiac production increases. The most significant effect with 94 elevated blood pressure–the' at your disposal' solution is that you'll require properly controlled drugs, both to combat your heart attack, to ensure that your bp doesn't go too far again, and to regulate your blood thinness. Regular blood checks will closely track the kidney and liver functions.

I am 70 years old. Is there anything else i would be given for my bp elevated because of my age?

Older individuals (those aged 65) have a higher risk of stroke or heart disease due to their age alone. Low-dose diuretics proved particularly useful for older people with elevated bp. An alternative is a blocker for the calcium-channel if thiazides cannot be provided. Very confusingly, a new large-scale clinical trial in the United States linked an ace inhibitor to a thiazide diuretic. In minimizing combined cardiovascular (stroke and heart attack) risks, the ace inhibitor was superior to a thiazide, with a comparable degree of decrease in bp. There is still some controversy about which type of bp-lowering medication is better for the primary care of older adults. Currently, the emphasis will be on strong bp regulation, regardless of the agent–thiazide, calcium-channel blocking, or ace inhibitor–is used.

Calcium-channel blockers should usually not be provided because you have a heart attack already.

2.2 Diabetes

I've had for a couple of years. I understand I'm at a higher risk of a heart attack or a stroke. What are the recommended treatments for someone who has diabetes and high bp?

Cardiovascular disorder mortality in individuals with both hypertension and diabetes hypertension and other conditions is elevated two-to three-fold relative to those of the general population. The mixture of diabetes and hypertension has, therefore, been branded as' double risk.' a lot of studies have shown that ace inhibitors, beta-blockers, and low-dose thiazide diuretics are effective in reducing this risk of dying from a heart attack or stroke.

If you have diabetes and high bp, you'll be treated as having mixed risk factors, and you'll be advised that blood sugar and bp levels are essential to monitoring. Your care should be stepped up to meet the optimal levels of bp, cholesterol, and blood sugar. Studies have shown that the goal of therapy is to decrease bp to below 130/80 mmHg, total cholesterol to below five mmol/liter, and glycosylated hemoglobin (long-acting sugar level indicator) to below 5%.

This is not necessary to ask whether an ace inhibitor, beta-blocker, or low-dose thiazide diuretic is used with your insulin in the treatment of your increased bp. Such medications have provided clinical trials with similar outcomes.

2.3 Kidney Problems

Recently I have had some kidney issues, and I'm concerned about needing to be screened for elevated bp now.

What Is It Going to Give Me?

It has been shown that ace inhibitors and angiotensin ii receptor antagonists decrease mortality from and development of kidney failure, and these medications should be the best ones for patients like yourself with elevated bp and kidney problems. Patients with diabetes (see issue above) continue to suffer from kidney complications as a potential risk to their diabetes, and many are diagnosed with ace inhibitors because they are more effective at trying to delay the development of kidney failure.

I was advised I had progressive kidney failure. What did you mean by that? I've always been informed I'm very likely to need medications that reduce bp. When, and what is it that they do?

Chronic kidney disease ('renal') may be categorized as a result of the reduced excretory activity (improper filtration of radioactive waste materials from the blood) or protein leakage from the urine. Both forms also overlap. High bp often occurs after these kinds of kidney problems, as the kidney plays a critical role in maintaining blood volume through the renin-angiotensin system. Diabetes is the most common reason for chronic renal failure, but other causes of chronic renal failure do occur.

When blood pressure tends to be high, end-stage renal failure can occur sooner, which includes dialysis. Furthermore, chronic kidney failure raises the risk of heart attack and stroke too.

There are two significant aspects of handling bp. First, it helps slow down renal failure, thereby reducing the risk of renal failure and dialysis at the end-stage. Third, it reduces increased cardiovascular risk.

Better regulation of bp, often with three or more medications to achieve target bp thresholds, is required to get these benefits.

Paradoxically, therapy with ace inhibitors and antagonists of the ace ii receptors can cause minor kidney problems. That suggests that if you have chronic kidney failure, you may be sent to a doctor for careful control of your renal function and drug therapy tailoring.

2.4 Increased Cholesterol Levels

I recently had a lipid check, and it was discovered that my cholesterol levels are significant. Will that be an issue in my high bp treatment?

Anomalies in lipid levels are often found in individuals with elevated bp.

These lead to an elevated risk of coronary hypertension along with other disease issues. Evidence also shows that the bp-reducing effects of medications such as diuretics and beta-blockers outweigh any potential changes in lipid profiles in individuals. So, therapy with thiazides and beta-blockers will also be prescribed as a first step, particularly in patients with elevated cholesterol rates.

How Can I Probably Be Given?

Statins are very effective in lowering blood cholesterol in LDL and VLDL.

Muscle cell inflammation ('myositis') has resulted in around 1 in 200 infected people, causing muscle discomfort, fatigue, or unexplained fever. Headache and liver injury are other potential side effects. Regular liver function screening is recommended for the first 15 months every six weeks and sometimes after that.

Statins are a new generation of cholesterol-lowering medications that are very effective and well-tolerated, launched in 1989.

Pravastatin (lip stat), atorvastatin (Lipitor), cerivastatin (lipobay), Fluvastatin (Lescol), and simvastatin (Zocor) are five drugs in this category so far. We act by inhibiting one enzyme involved in the synthesis of cholesterol.

Statins are highly effective medications for those with coronary heart disease and those without it.

New randomized statin studies in people with elevated bp (who have not had a heart attack in the past) have found that the risk of a fatal or non-fatal heart attack has been decreased from 5% to 3% over five years. For women, the advantages of statins could well be more moderate at reducing these risks. Recent wisdom is that patients with mildly elevated cholesterol levels should have their risk measured, and their care for bp and cholesterol will be determined in the light of this test.

2.5 Problems Requiring Beta or Alpha-Blockers

I have extreme asthma and conditions involving beta-or alpha-blockers, and my doctor will not put me on beta-blockers despite my elevated bp. How will such medications in people with asthma be avoided?

Beta-blockers improve inflammation of the airways in persons with known or latent asthma. However, because the beta-blockers have various effects on the airways (known as' selective' or' non-selective beta-blockers'), certain forms of beta-blockers are more dangerous than others. Some persons with chronic bronchitis or emphysema often have unrecognized asthma. There have been deaths from the use of beta-blockers in these patients, and the doctor should test airway resistance with someone with some sort of weak chest before initiating the beta-blockers.

Most frequently than not, alternate bp-lowering agents are available and can be used in these cases.

Generally speaking, selective beta-blocker agents are preferred to non-selective agents, i.e., drugs which function only on the heart rather than on the airways of the lungs. In people with asthma or obstructive disease of the airways, non-selective beta-blockers have to be prevented. Selective beta-blockers can be used in some instances where effective bp-lowering medications are not available or where obstructive inflammation of the airways can only be marginally enhanced.

Each month I suffer from migraines. I am now sick with massive bp. Is this going to impact which medications I get prescribed?

Beta-blockers are used to prevent a migraine attack from arising. These are usually recommended by those suffering from migraines and high bp for this cause, and you should typically be given these first to see if you get on.

I was given beta-blockers for my high bp and later found I was having real trouble making my wife love.

Will it be the drugs that caused my erection problems? Was there anything else I could get for the bp?

You are right. Beta-blockers are concerned with problems with orgasm but to a lesser degree than diuretic ones. It is felt by as many as 15–20 percent of people who take high-dose diuretics (e.g., 5 mg bendrofluazide). When you have issues with this area, see the doctor fix them as other medications are going to be recommended, too.

I have prostate signs. Were there a few bp-lowering medications more appropriate for me?

Drugs blocking the alpha-adrenoceptor have the benefit of reducing bp while at the same time, relieving the effects of prostate obstruction.

Alpha-blocker trials, however, were not healthy, evidently raising the risk of heart failure. When you suffer from heart disease, they are not given. The specialist will determine whether new kinds of medications are available.

2.6 Blood-Thinning Drugs

I was advised to take a small dose of aspirin a day, blood-thinning medications, but I still take high bp medications for my bp. Is there any risk that I should take aspirin because I do have elevated bp?

Aspirin is a drug that has many benefits — mostly by minimizing the chance of stroke and heart attack — but is often fraught with adverse effects, typically causing damage to the stomach. Patients at high risk of stroke or heart disease (usually taken 5 percent over five years) generally are receiving considerably more benefit than aspirin damage. When you are on non-100 high blood pressure, the steroidal anti-inflammatory medications at your disposal' guide, the chance of suffering from such bleeding will be more elevated, and both can be stopped when necessary. Speak to the doctor about your issues–when considering the topic of care for high bp, you will also warn the doctor that you are taking other medications.

You can speak to a different doctor than usual, and he or she will not be aware of the other problems.

Anticoagulants like warfarin or heparin are recommended by physicians almost exclusively. Then you can't help because those who do recommend them will still test the need for aspirin.

2.7 Racial Variations

My family originally came from Jamaica, and my dad has a high bp. It is running in our household. Will black people differ from white people in the way they react to drugs that deplete bp?

Black people from African Caribbean countries are especially at risk of experiencing high bp. High bp also appears to be more serious, with an increased risk of complications, including stroke and kidney failure.

In this group of people, non-drug therapy, particularly salt cutting, tends to be more successful.

So far as opioid addiction is concerned, indeed, people of African Caribbean origin react less well to beta-blocker drugs and ace inhibitors, because this category suppresses the renin-angiotensin mechanism. It has been shown they respond to thiazide diuretics and calcium-channel blockers better than other ethnic groups.

Additionally, people with a southern Asian heritage are more likely to develop elevated rates of bp and diabetes, especially at risk of developing coronary heart disease.

Yet their reaction to bp-lowering drugs is close to that of white European-born men. Asians need to be especially vigilant of their risk of coronary heart failure, and hypertension with other complications also benefit from treatment with aspirin and statin as well as their bp medicine.

2.8 Pain–Particularly Joint Pain and Arthritis

I have to move on to high bp pills but do have arthritis and take ibuprofen for pain. Can my arthritis diagnosis impact whether I am prescribed for high bp?

Joint pains are typically caused by osteoarthritis or reactive arthritis, most often caused by rheumatoid arthritis. Treatment is generally achieved with an anti-inflammatory non-steroidal drug (NSAID).

Most of these medications are available, with some — such as ibuprofen (brufen, fenbid) — now available at chemists around the counter.

Both NSAIDs appear to be effective in treating reactive arthritis and gout. Their effect is generally dramatic in acute gout. These can benefit osteoarthritis patients, but their impact is typically less drastic. These are also used in the treatment of period pains and severe menstrual blood loss ('menorrhagia'), and particularly mefenamic acid (ponstan) has been promoted for this reason.

Many NSAIDs increase bp by an average diastolic pressure of 5-6 mmHg, approximately the same as the decrease that most bp-decreasing medications achieve. We do tend to induce accumulation of salt.

Approximately 40 percent of the patients who require bp-lowering medications often suffer from chronic rheumatic pain and are frequently prescribed NSAIDs.

You need to be aware of the effect of NSAIDs on your bp and ask for an alternate medication from your doctor–paracetamol, which is not a NSAID, will offer excellent pain relief without any of the side effects on bp rise. Ibuprofen, sold over the counter, has a much smaller impact than most other NSAIDs and is less than two mmHg on average. If the drug you are buying is likely to affect your bp or interact with your bp-lowering medications, you should ask a pharmacist.

I have the ultimate antidepressant (prednisolone) diagnosis of rheumatoid arthritis. Was this going to affect my elevated bp treatment?

Steroidal medications (usually in the form of prednisone or adrenocorticotrophic hormone-acth) are essential and useful for severe, acute rheumatoid arthritis attacks, particularly in the first few months after the onset of the disease. They can ease not only pain in these situations but also mitigate long-term joint injury. Because they increase bp by inducing accumulation of salt and sodium, and therefore increasing blood pressure, this is almost always a price worth paying, particularly for those with extremely high bp.

In either case, these extreme cases should typically be under the care of a medical specialist, whose role is to make an informed judgment in the light of all the facts in your situation.

Long-term use of rheumatoid arthritis drugs not only increases bp (seldom by too much) but also weakens the bone system with a high risk of accidental spine breaks, which decreases respiratory capacity and susceptibility to all sorts of infections. There are different disease-modifying medicines available so that you can inquire about them to the gp or expert.

Rheumatologists usually hold drugs off patients with rheumatoid arthritis for as long as possible. Raised bp is one of the lower long-term drug risks, even in individuals with elevated bp.

I've had many gout attacks in the past, and now I'm taking medications that are dropping bp. Many forms of bp-lowering medications I have been advised can induce gout. Is that real, then?

Gout happens when the body is not getting rid of any of its waste materials, a drug called uric acid.

The kidneys usually get rid of the uric acid in your blood, so it's flushed out in your urine.

You have a metabolic disorder in your developing gout, and too much uric acid is formed and deposited as crystals in your body's joints. It will lead to extreme discomfort, inflammation, redness, and tenderness of the infected joint, the big toe joint most frequently. It's a big concern that appears to run in households.

Alcohol, certain foods (liver is a good example), and high-dosage thiazide diuretics can increase uric acid levels in your blood. There is barely any effect on uric acid levels at low doses (usually 2.5 mg of bendrofluazide daily), and little impact at 1,25 mg at all. Equally effective in controlling bp are such small doses. Gout was a significant concern with people taking high-dose thiazides, but the side effect of gout is much less severe because the bp-lowering results can be obtained with low-dose thiazides.

There is some evidence that higher dose thiazide diuretics increase the chance of gout recurrence in individuals who continue to suffer from gout (past diagnosis or family history). So, you won't be given thiazide diuretics–substitute bp-lowering medications are recommended.

2.9 Psychological Problems

My mother has acquired schizophrenia, but she still has high bp. Can her hypertension disorder affect what she is treated for?

Most patients with schizophrenia are typically diagnosed with prescription tranquilizer medications-phenothiazine-usually once a month as capsules or depot injections. Such medications have a robust bp-lowering effect, which is usually inappropriate with any other bp-lowering treatment.

Involuntary writhing motions, typically of the face and extremities, are a typical complication of long-term phenothiazine therapy. Methyldopa (Aldomet) improves this effect, and it cannot be used to treat elevated bp in people with schizophrenia.

Chapter 3: Medication and Blood Pressure

3.1 High Blood Pressure Medications and Their Roles

1. Diuretics Made from Thiazide.

Diuretics, also called water tablets, are drugs that work on the kidneys to help extract salt and water from the bloodstream, lowering blood flow.

Thiazide diuretics are often the only, but not the only, option of drugs for elevated blood pressure. Diuretics of thiazide include chlorthalidone, hydrochlorothiazide (Microzide), and others.

If you are not taking a diuretic and your blood pressure remains high, talk to your doctor about adding one or replacing a diuretic medication you are currently taking. In people of African descent and older people, diuretics or calcium channel blockers can function better than angiotensin-converting enzyme (ace) inhibitors alone. An intensified urination is a typical side effect of the diuretics.

2. Enzyme-Converting Angiotensin (Ace) Inhibitors.

Such drugs— such as lisinopril (Zestril), benazepril (Lotensin), captopril (Capoten), and others— tend to open blood vessels by preventing the development of a natural chemical that narrows the blood vessels. People with chronic kidney disease may get the advantage of using one of their drugs as an ace inhibitor.

3. Blockers of the Angiotensin Ii Receptors (Arbs).

Such drugs tend to open blood vessels by blocking the action of a natural chemical that narrows the blood arteries, not the shape.

Candesartan (Atacand), losartan (Cozaar), and others are found in arb. Persons with chronic kidney disease can benefit as one of their drugs from getting an arb.

4. Signal Blocks for Calcium.

These drugs— like amlodipine (Norvasc), diltiazem (Cardizem, Tiazac, others), and so on— help calm the blood vessel muscles. Your heart rate is slowing some. In older people and people of African descent, calcium channel blockers can function better than ace inhibitors do alone.

Grapefruit juice combines with other antagonists of the calcium receptor, increasing blood levels of the drug, and placing you at a higher risk for side effects. If you are worried about the experiences, speak to the doctor or pharmacist.

3.2 Other Medicines Often Used to Treat High Blood Pressure

If you have difficulty meeting your blood pressure goal with a combination of the above medication, your doctor can prescribe: • alpha-blockers.

Such medications reduce blood vessel nerve signals, reducing the effects of natural chemicals that widen the blood vessels. Alpha-blockers include doxazosin (Cardura), Minipress (prazosin), and others.

• Blockers of Alpha-Beta.

Alpha-beta blockers pause the heartbeat and decrease the volume of blood that needs to be pumped into the arteries, in addition to minimizing nervous impulses through blood vessels. Blockers for the alpha-beta include carvedilol (Coreg) and labetalol (Trandate).

• Blockers in Beta.

Such medications lower the pressure on your heart and open your blood vessels, allowing the heart to pump more steadily and with less energy. Acebutolol (Sectral), atenolol (Tenormin), among others, are beta-blockers.

Beta-blockers are typically not used as the only drug you are given, but they may be beneficial when paired with other medications for blood pressure.

- Antagonisms of Aldosterone.

Types include spironolactone (Aldactone) and inspire (eplerenone). Such medications inhibit the influence of natural chemicals, which can lead to the accumulation of salt and sodium, which can add to elevated blood pressure.

- Inhibitors of the Renin

Aliskiren (tekturna) slows down renin development, an enzyme the kidneys generate that starts a series of chemical steps that raise blood pressure.

Aliskiren works by reducing the renin's ability to continue the cycle. You should not be taking aliskiren with ace inhibitors or arbs due to a risk of serious complications, including stroke.

- Vasodilator.

These medicines, including hydralazine and minoxidil, work directly on the muscles in the walls of your arteries, preventing tightening of muscles and narrowing of your arteries.

- Agents Key to Policy.

Such medications block your brain from controlling your nervous system to increase your heart rate and widen your blood vessels. Guanfacine like Intuniv, Tenex, Clonidine (Catapres, kapvay), and methyldopa are examples of this.

Your doctor can recommend a mixture of low-dose medicines rather than larger doses of a single medication to minimize the number of daily doses you need. Also, two or three drugs for blood pressure are sometimes more effective than one. It is often a matter of trial and error to determine the most appropriate prescription or a combination of medications.

3.3 Resistant Hypertension:

When your blood pressure is impossible to regulate, you might have resistant hypertension because your blood pressure stays stubbornly elevated after having at least three different forms of high blood pressure medications, all of which would usually be a diuretic all.

Individuals who have managed elevated blood pressure but at the same time take four different forms of drugs are often known to have resistant hypertension to maintain such control. The likelihood of high blood pressure being a secondary factor will usually be reconsidered.

Having immune hypertension doesn't mean you'll never drop your blood pressure. If you and your doctor can understand what's causing your persistently elevated blood pressure, there's a strong possibility you can reach your target with the aid of more successful care.

Your doctor or expert in hypertension may: evaluate possible causes of your condition to decide whether they can be treated check medications you are taking for specific disorders to suggest that you should not take any medicines that aggravate your blood pressure ensure that you check your blood pressure at home and see whether you will have elevated blood pressure in your doctor's office (white coat hypertension)

When you do not take your medicines for high blood pressure precisely as prescribed, then your blood pressure can pay the price. When you miss doses because you can't afford the drugs, because you have adverse effects or fail to take the narcotics, speak to the doctor for remedies. Should not change the care without advice from the specialist.

3.4 Vitamin Supplement Recommendations

For vitamins and minerals as well as micronutrients. Not all vitamins are equivalent when it comes to the treatment of blood pressure. These heart-healthy vitamin recommendations can help lower your blood pressure.

A dosage notes: we used iu (international units), milligrams, and micrograms to denote similar doses. Not all doses in milligrams are given in iu since the effectiveness of various vitamins varies. For in, 100 iu of vitamin a may not be equal to 100 iu of vitamin d.

Vitamin A

You learn that eating carrots that are high in vitamin a (beta carotene) prevents vision loss. Vitamin A also clears the blood of free radicals and can also play a part in the prevention of heart disease.

Vitamin B

Vitamin b functions with vitamin b12 and vitamin c in the production of red blood cells. It can also help to lower certain people's high blood pressure. One possible way to reduce folic acid blood pressure is by decreasing elevated homocysteine levels in people suffering from high blood pressure.

You can easily have the recommended daily amount of folic acid in your diet by consuming beans, peanuts and legumes, citrus fruit, dark green leafy vegetables, poultry, pork, shellfish, and liver. Adequate levels of folic acid are especially essential in some classes, such as women of childbearing age.

Vitamin C

Vitamin c is an antioxidant that can play a role in cancer control. Clinically, vitamin c has been thought to alleviate symptoms of high blood pressure potentially, but it has not yet been shown to regulate heart disease.

Aside from citrus fruits and juices, healthy food sources of vitamin c include bananas, sweet red peppers, onions, and potatoes.

Vitamin D

Research shows that increasing the dose of vitamin d, which regulates the body's metabolism and adjust phosphorus and calcium level in the blood, can reduce blood pressure. Blood vessels and the heart have a large number of vitamin d receptors, meaning that vitamin D plays a role in cardiovascular health.Especially vitamin D3.

Although I can't assume that vitamin d deficiency leads to high blood pressure, people with a low amount of vitamin d are more likely to develop cardiovascular disease. Studies show that low vitamin d levels associated with high blood pressure almost double the risk of myocardial infarction, stroke, and heart failure.

That said, access to sunlight and the intake of vitamin d-rich foods is the best bet on your daily dose of vitamin d. Blood pressure increases as the exposure to sunlight decreases. Fifteen minutes of sun exposure (natural or sunlight) per day gives you a generous dose of vitamin d. Salmon, milk, eggs, mushrooms, tuna, and vitamin d enriched flour and baked goods are all excellent dietary sources of this vitamin.

Make sure you know how much vitamin d you need because excess vitamin d can cause toxic build-up in the body. For example, people between 50 and 70 years of age need more than younger peers and may also gain more from additional blood pressure doses.

Vitamin E

Vitamin e (d-alpha tocopherol) is an antioxidant with vitamins a and c. While vitamin e may decrease the risk of cancer and heart disease, it does not appear to be the case at the moment. However, not all vitamin e is equal. Many nutritionists agree that the natural source of vitamin e is safer than the synthetic version (dl-alpha tocopherol). As a result, taking significant quantities of vitamin e capsules (as with any vitamin) is dangerous.

Some studies have proposed that the incremental rise in the dose of vitamin e decreases blood pressure slowly and safely, but this has not yet been confirmed.

Most Americans get enough vitamin e from dietary sources, but people on low-fat diets will need supplementation. There are claims that vitamin e will potentially cause a rise in blood pressure if it is taken in excess. The US institute of medicine recommends 1,000 milligrams per day (equivalent to 1,500 iu) as the maximum upper limit dosage for additional alpha-tocopherol.

Most adult males and females will consume vitamin e via diet, and supplementation is generally not required. Good sources of vitamin e include vegetable oils, sesame seeds, sunflower seeds, whole grain bread, cereals and pasta, nuts, spinach, broccoli, mangoes, kiwi, egg yolks and wheat germs.

Vitamin K

Vitamin k, a fat-soluble vitamin, is also known as potassium. This book discusses its role in the control of blood pressure.

Some evidence indicates that vitamin k could be more active as an antioxidant and anti-high blood pressure micronutrient than vitamin e or even coenzyme q10. Vitamin k assists in neuron activity, maintain a healthy heart rate and blood pressure, prevents blood clots, and promotes muscle contractions. Pregnant women may need higher doses. Also, some antibiotics may lead to a deficiency of vitamin [262], bringing down high blood pressure k. Using caution if you are taking an anticoagulant (anti-blood clot) drug.

Zinc

Several drugs that are ostensibly designed to reduce blood pressure contain zinc. This mineral is an antioxidant that battles cardiovascular diseases and prevents free radicals. It helps maintain adequate levels of vitamin e in the blood and helps reduce blood pressure and controls blood flow. Zinc will also reduce the high blood pressure caused by too much cadmium. Not much zinc is required to keep your blood pressure down. Good sources of zinc are meat, poultry, fish, eggs, nuts, seeds, and grains.

Selenium

Low levels of selenium are associated with cardiovascular disease, as selenium helps control blood flow and clears the blood of cadmium, a mineral that raises blood pressure. Selenium is used to cleanse the blood of free radicals and to preserve a balanced heart and blood vessels. You will increase your selenium by eating Brazil nuts, whole grains, and shellfish.

Phosphorus

Phosphorus interacts with other minerals to reduce blood pressure.

Beware: too much phosphorus can lead to increased cardiac deaths in patients with chronic kidney disease or pre-heart disease. Adults aged 70 and over will reduce the amount of phosphorus intake.

Healthy dietary phosphorus sources include milk and dairy products, dried peas, beans, and lentils as well as nuts and seeds

3.5 Effectiveness of Weight Management While Elevating Blood Pressure Problems

The association between overweight or obese and blood pressure and risk of hypertension is good. A strong correlation between body weight and blood pressure was observed in men as early as the 1920s. 13, 14, this relationship has been consistently verified by epidemiological research in the intervening years. The Framingham study showed that hypertension is almost twice as common in the obese of both sexes.15 Stamler and colleagues16 observed a risk ratio of 2.42 for younger adults compared to nonobese hypertension (BMI of less than 25) and 1.54 for older people. The nurse's health study17 compared people with BMI of less than 22 to those over 29 and observed a 2-to6-fold hypertension prevalence in obese women.

More recent Framingham report results further reinforce this relationship. Framingham participants from both sexes, separated into quintiles of BMI, showed higher blood pressure with decreased overweight. In this case, those in the most top BMI quintile exhibited higher systolic pressure of 16 mm hg and higher diastolic blood pressure of 9 mm hg than those in the lowest quintile.

It translates into an improvement of 4 mm hg for each 4.5 kg of elevated weight with systolic blood pressure.18 in younger Canadian adults, rabkin et al19 observed a 5-fold higher occurrence of hypertension in people with bmis of more than 30 compared with those with less than 20 for both sexes.

The effect of hypertension on public health is still immense. Although perhaps impossible to pick out due to correlations with other risk factors, including overweight, hypertension is a significant contributor to most chronic disease categories.20 heart disease and cerebrovascular disorder are the first and third significant causes of death in the United States. Twenty-one hypertensions are one of the cleanest reasons of death in the United States. With the safe people 2010 plan, the federal government is aiming to raise those in the adult hypertensive population with managed hypertension to 50 percent.22 that compares with the presently projected 34 percent. Eight blood pressure management, the restoration of blood pressure to normotensive level, will have a direct effect on cardiac and cerebrovascular mortality.

In clinical trials, antihypertensive treatment will lead to a decrease in the rate of stroke, myocardial infarction, and heart failure of between 20% and 50%.23 Ogden et al2 suggest that a 12-mm drop in systolic blood pressure sustained in a population with initial stage 1 hypertension over ten years would reduce accident mortality by between 9% and 11%.

A population-wide improvement of 5.5 mm hg systolic or 3.0 mm hg diastolic will result in an estimated 15 percent decline in coronary heart attack events and a 27 percent decline in stroke.24, 25 thus, the question is how to accomplish this goal.

Numerous therapies have proved successful in potentially dramatically reducing blood pressure levels, at least in the near term.8 of these, weight loss provides a variety of desirable characteristics.

They must find the findings of weight loss induced blood pressure improvements achieved by the more conventional methods of dietary control and other lifestyle modification techniques. We do not review the weight loss data resulting from pharmacological or surgical procedures except where it can apply to weight loss maintenance

Alteration of blood pressure is theorized as being directly linked to weight increase. Although several studies have examined this from a perspective of weight loss and reduction in blood pressure, there are few data in humans to directly inform the idea that weight gain relates to high blood pressure at the individual level. Animal experiments were the primary source of knowledge. Rocchini ET al26 observed substantial changes in blood pressure that would follow weight gain from dog overfeeding. Hall ET al27 confirmed the relationship.

On the other hand, numerous human clinical interventions have examined the relationship between weight loss and changes in blood pressure. Haynes28 analyzed six clinical trials available at the time related to weight loss and blood pressure, stating the 3 of them had a substantial weight loss effect. In contrast, the other 3 had no apparent impact. More recently, neter et al. 29 conducted a meta-analysis of 25 studies on this subject. The authors found that a 1-kg body weight loss was correlated with an estimated 1-mm hg decrease in blood pressure. Further, this decrease in blood pressure was achieved without the need to reach a healthy weight status as well. Some of the biggest of such trials, the test of hypertension prevention (tohp), included a weight loss control arm.30

In this case, a weight loss of 2 kg over six months resulted in a reduction of 3.7 mm hg in systolic and 2.7 mm hg in diastolic blood pressure.

A decrease of 42 percent was observed in this study in the case of hypertension.31 how overweight, and blood pressure functions physiologically due to the existing correlation between weight shift and blood pressure levels, the question arises as to whether this relationship works physiologically. Rocchini33 discusses various possible biological pathways by which weight loss or fat loss may contribute to concurrent blood pressure declines. These include reductions in insulin resistance, increased sodium retention, changes in vascular structure and function, changes in ion transport, increased stimulation of the renin--system, increased activation of the sympathetic nervous system, and changes in the natriuretic peptide. The wide variety of alternative pathways can also be a significant factor in accounting for the perceived variability of the reaction to any therapy of blood pressure. Weight loss can affect one or more of these proposed routes of action variable and simultaneously. Since weight status itself is the product of several factors, it wouldn't necessarily differ how it produces changes in blood pressure.

Increasing activity to lose weight if your doctor recommends weight loss, there's an easy rule to follow, which is to move more, eat less, and make smarter food choices. Slowly increase your physical exercise level above the 150-minute aha guideline of moderate-intensity aerobic activity, lessen the number of calories you take, and consume a balanced diet. After you have achieved your target weight, you will then decide which food and exercise options work well to keep your weight going.

The two key reasons for keeping a healthy weight are:

- Eating well
- Walking regularly

When you intend to lose weight, explore a balanced solution with your healthcare provider.

For one, the doctor will help you find out how much calories you need to lose weight and instruct you about the right types of activities.

Chapter 4: Supplement and Exercise

4.1 One Move That Helps Lower Your Blood Pressure without Medication

Getting just a little more active every day is known to help lower your blood pressure and hold it down. And walking is an entirely free, safe, and simple way to achieve that goal.

Walking has a positive impact on your overall wellbeing, but is especially effective at helping you regulate your blood pressure.

Holding the blood pressure in a safe range is considered to be one of the most potent ways to prevent a host of illnesses, including heart disease and stroke. And doing a simple workout like walking is known to be a perfect drug-free way to maintain healthy blood pressure or help bring it down if it's still high.

And why is it that as many as 75 million of us — one in three people, according to the centers for disease control and prevention — have high blood pressure at the moment, sometimes without even realizing it?

The cause is simple: high blood pressure (also referred to as HBP or hypertension) typically has no symptoms. This doesn't cause chest pain, for example, or make you bounce and buff when ascending the stairs. The American heart association recommendations describe blood pressure as usual at less than 120/80 millimeters of mercury (mmHg) and high blood pressure at 140/90 mmHg or higher.

If you find out that your blood pressure is going in the wrong direction, there is good news: only small amounts of physical exercise will help keep your blood pressure in check or lower if it is still higher than it should be.

4.2 Can Low-Intensity Exercise Like Walking Reduce Your Blood Pressure?

Sure, sure. For a seminal study for menopause, researchers at the Pennington biomedical research center in Baton Rouge, Louisiana, surveyed about 400 people between the ages of 45 and 75. They were both overweight and obese, sedentary, and had high blood pressure. Researchers divided the women into four classes, three of which had different strength rates and lengths of time. The fourth group has remained sedentary.

Six months later, all three classes of involved women had higher blood pressure rates. The figures for the group that performed the most rigorous workout were just marginally higher than the statistics of the group that did the least intensive job. While women did not lose weight, they benefited greatly from enhancing their cardiovascular fitness.

Regular exercise also helps to relieve stress by reining stress hormones in the body, including cortisol, states Harvard health. It is important because stress can raise blood pressure even in young adults, according to research published online on 28 October 2016 in frontiers in psychology.

4.3 How Much Exercise Do You Need to Keep Your Blood Pressure Under Control?

Ideally, everyone— but particularly those with medical conditions such as type 2 diabetes, heart disease, and high blood pressure— should have at least two and a half hours of moderate exercise per week, says cardiologist Tracy Stevens, MD, of the saint Luke mid-America heart institute in Kansas City, Missouri.

"try for at least 30 minutes a day most days of the week, and never go for more than two days without any workout," says Dr. Stevens, who is also a professor of medicine at Missouri University in Kansas City. "Walking is one of the safest and simplest activities that you can do. You can walk anywhere, so there's no need for any gear beyond a decent pair of sneakers. "if you're frustrated by the prospect of participating in a fitness routine, relax. What you have to do is start walking for just five minutes, three times a day, Stevens says. Such fast walks will be more rapid every time, which, in effect, will make it easier to keep walking a little longer. Before you know it, the first 5 minutes will be 6, then 8, then 10 — and doing 10 minutes three times a day will add up to the 30 minutes you need.

Another way to get going is by slipping a few fast bursts of exercise into your day. Small moves that can add up include parking a little further from the doorway everywhere you go — to work, to the grocery store, to the doctor's appointments bringing the grocery stores in your car one bag at a time planning meals and running around the kitchen while you cook instead of ordering taking-off. Use stairs rather than the elevator if you're going up or down one or two flights walking down the stairs. One right choice is to walk in a heated swimming pool; warm water will soothe and relax rather than stress joints. A recumbent cycle could be another reasonable option, says Stevens. It is wise to talk to your doctor about your workout schedule, who will give your personal advice.

4.4 What Will Make It Easier to Stick to A Daily Exercise?

You are taking your blood pressure before and after the workout. "the effects of exercise for reducing blood pressure are so drastic that it's a perfect motivator," says Stevens.

Exercise every day at the same time. It's going to become a part of the routine, making it harder to miss.

Carry comfortable shoes, please. When you work out outside, dress up for the weather — choose light fabrics that you can take off while you work up a sweat.

Meet a fellow exercise man. When anyone else is counting on you, you won't want to let them down. And a good chat makes time quicker.

Just make it fun. As we all know, when the task is enjoyable, we're more likely to repeat it. So, make sure you choose hobbies that you enjoy and mix things up regularly to prevent boredom. Walking is fine, but so are walking, hula-hooping, swimming, ice-skating, cycling, and tag-playing.

4.5 The 6 Best Exercises to Reduce High Blood Pressure

Do you need to lower your blood pressure by up to 20 points? One of the easiest ways to achieve so is by returning to your healthy body weight. You can measure this by setting the body mass index (use the BMI calculator at the bottom of the page).

To help you hit your weight goal and help lower your blood pressure in the process, find these six exercises/activities, says Wesley Tyree, MD, a cardiologist and an active member of the HonorHealth medical staff:

1. Walking

Ten minutes of fast or moderate walking three times a day lowers blood pressure by reducing the stiffness of the blood vessels so that blood can flow more easily. The results of exercise are most apparent during and directly after workouts. Lower blood pressure may be the most important thing right after you work out.

Therefore, health experts theorize, the best way to combat high blood pressure could be to break up the exercise in a few sessions during the day. One study showed that three 10-minute walks a day more effectively reduced potential blood pressure spikes than one 30-minute trek a day.

2. Running

Thirty minutes a day of running or stationary cycling or three 10-minute stretches of cycling, the same logic applies here as for walking.

3. Hiking

The muscle strength you need to climb a path on a slope, a hill, or a mountain will help you reach a higher level of fitness. Physical exercise, such as walking, can reduce blood pressure by up to 10 points.

4. Desk treadmills or pedals driving

Blood pressure levels were even more ideal in the test when the participants blew up at a slow speed of1-mile-per-hour at desk-based treadmills for at least 10 minutes per hour or pedaled stationary bikes under the desk for at least 10 minutes per hour.

5. Weight training

While it sounds counter-intuitive, weight training or lifting can reduce blood pressure. Strength training often increases blood pressure levels slightly, which can also boost general health, which also improves blood pressure levels.

6. Swimming

This type of exercise can help manage blood pressure in adults 60 years of age and older, another study found. Throughout 12 weeks, the swimmer-participants slowly trained for up to 45 minutes of continuous swimming at a time. By the conclusion of the test, the swimmers had reduced their systolic blood pressure by an average of nine points.

"The advantages of exercise are not understood if exercise is not continued," dr. Tyree said, "and the' use it or lose it' principle is valid. You will lose gains after stopping exercise for two weeks. Moderate exercise for 150 minutes per week or intense exercise for 75 minutes per week is the standard recommendation."

4.6 Supplements to Lower Blood Pressurevist

Many people are interested in using naturopathy.

Before beginning any medication to treat high blood pressure, you should first consult with your doctor. Supplements on their own cannot be enough to overcome high blood pressure.

1. Folic Acid

The increased volume of blood due to pregnancy can lead to high blood pressure.

Folic acid is an essential aid to the growth of a baby in the womb. Studies show that folic acid can have the added advantage of reducing the risk of hypertension during pregnancy.

High doses of folic acid can also help to lower blood pressure significantly in both men and women with high blood pressure, as seen in the 2009 trusted source meta-analysis.

The dose of folic acid, which is in most prenatal vitamins, but it can also be obtained as a separate supplement and taken in capsule form.

2. Vitamin D

Low vitamin d levels have been related to hypertension by a reliable source. However, the authoritative source clinical review of 11 studies found that vitamin d supplements had a minimal effect on diastolic blood pressure and had no effect on systolic blood pressure in people with high blood pressure.

While it is necessary to have sufficient vitamin d, its effects on high blood pressure can be minimal.

You can buy vitamin d capsules anywhere supplements are available. You should also increase the amount of vitamin d in your diet and spend time out to absorb vitamin d through your skin.

3. Magnesium

Your body uses mineral magnesium to control healthy cell activity. Magnesium also helps with muscle fiber contractions.

Several reports are unclear as to whether magnesium helps relieve blood pressure. Nevertheless, one study of trusted sources found that magnesium supplements can have a minor impact on blood pressure.

Magnesium supplements are available online and in natural food stores.

4. Potassium

Potassium helps to reduce the influence of sodium on blood pressure. The American heart association also says that potassium helps to minimize the stress on the artery walls. Studies endorse potassium supplementation as a treatment for reducing blood pressure.

Potassium supplements can be sold in natural food stores and online. The average dosage is 99 milligrams (mg) a day.

5. Coq10 Coenzyme

Q10 (also known as ubiquinone) is an antioxidant that helps the cells generate energy. In a clinical trial study of a reliable source, coq10 lowered diastolic blood pressure by up to 10 millimeters of mercury (mm hg) and systolic blood pressure by 17 mm hg.

Coq10 is commonly considered healthy and can be purchased in capsule form. Check it out here.

6. Fiber

Dietary fiber levels in the traditional western diet tend to be much lower than recommended. Increasing your fiber intake may prevent hypertension or lower blood pressure if you already have it.

A trusted source was found to reduce blood pressure by a small amount in the study of clinical trials with a fiber supplement of 11 grams a day.

You can also add more fiber to your diet by growing your intake of green, leafy vegetables and fresh fruits. You will find one here if you want to take a supplement.

7. Acetyl-L-Carnitine

Acetyl-l-carnitine (alcar) is used by the body to generate electricity. It's made in your body, but it can also be purchased as a supplement. Alcar is a promising option to regulate blood pressure. Most people are free, inexpensive, and well-tolerated.

While not much work has been done to support its use for high blood pressure, a small study indicated that it could help to reduce systolic blood pressure.

L-carnitine supplements can be found here for purchase.

8. Garlic

Garlic has been used as a diuretic and circulatory remedy since ancient Greece.

Garlic will change the way your body circulates blood through your system. This, therefore, makes sense because, when tested, trusted source substantially reduced both diastolic and systolic blood pressure in randomized clinical trials.

Both garlic supplements and raw garlic can be used to assist with high blood pressure.

9. Melatonin

Melatonin is a hormone that is released by our body. It's most often linked to helping you sleep. Persons with hypertension often may not generate enough melatonin. Researchers have found that taking melatonin supplements may help reduce the blood pressure of trusted source.

You should consider taking 2 mg of melatonin as a healthy, uncommon way to reduce your blood pressure at night. It's not advised to take it in the afternoon, because it can make you sleepy.

Melatonin is available in liquid and capsule form.

10. Omega-3s from fish oil or linseed supplements

Omega-3 fatty acids help your body boost your cardiovascular tone. It makes omega-3 a valuable ingredient for reducing blood pressure.

One analysis of the literature on omega-3s and blood pressure concluded that omega-3 supplements reduced blood pressure' slightly, but significantly, trusted source.' omega-3s are present in fish oil supplements as well as linseed supplements (capsules and liquids). Check out this final beginner's guide to omega-3 fatty acids if this is a new supplement for you.

11. Anthocyanins

Anthocyanins are red, purple, or blue pigments present in certain fruits and vegetables. Cherry, pomegranate, blueberry, and other antioxidant-rich fruits contain anthocyanins.

This component may be the reason why pomegranate juice performed in a 2004 study to reduce systolic blood pressure by 12 percent over a year. In another study, however, anthocyanins appeared to have little effect on blood pressure.

Most foods, such as elderberry or acai extract, contain anthocyanins— though not all of them have been clearly shown to affect blood pressure.

If you're interested in finding out about it, check out your nearest health food store or buy elderberry supplements here.

12. French maritime bark extract

French marine bark extract is a dietary supplement that uses the antioxidant strength of flavonoids.

Pycnogenol, derived from French marine bark, can improve circulation and help lower blood pressure. Participants in a clinical study took 125 mg Pycnogenol daily for 12 weeks and had significant benefits.

Takeaway herbal supplements are a safe way of treating high blood pressure. But certain drugs can interfere with blood pressure medications, such as ace inhibitors and beta-blockers.

If you are still taking blood pressure drugs, speak to your doctor about potential complications and risk alerts before you try a replacement.

It is essential to know that most supplements have been shown to reduce blood pressure modestly. When you have been diagnosed with high blood pressure, a supplement may help — but it may not reduce enough blood pressure on its own.

Important note:

Several blood pressures drugs have also been shown to minimize heart attacks, strokes, and death from heart disease. Although several supplements can help to lower blood pressure slightly, they have not been shown to reduce the risk of heart attacks and strokes in people with high blood pressure. Please make sure to speak to your doctor about the appropriate care options for your particular needs.

If buying supplements, note that the food and drug administration does not monitor them in the same way as prescription drugs are. Just buy supplements from suppliers you trust.

Chapter 5: Dealing with Blood Pressure in Daily Life

5.1 Which Diet Is Best?

By the end of the day, the right diet is the one you can stay with long enough not just to shed weight but also to alter and strengthen your eating habits. It won't do any good to lose the extra pounds just to win them back with a couple more; this type of yo-yo diet potentially hurts the body.

While there were hundreds of diet books, many of which entered the best-seller list, they all fell into one or another category. You may have tried one of those diets, or more.

• Gimmick diets allow you to focus on one item or another (grapefruit or cabbage soup diets), never mix foods of various types at a time (fit for life and others), mix foods in a very particular manner (zone diet and others), alternate foods during the week, splurge after "doing healthy" for a few days, or do some form of fasting.

The next time you're tempted to try one of those fad diets, ask yourself if you can imagine eating that way in your life.

• Low-carb diets pledge you will consume all the fatty foods you love, from steak to bacon to butter, but most carbohydrate-containing foods will be omitted. The Atkins diet the most famous of these, although they've been around in one incarnation or another for decades. As mouthwatering as this approach, no matter how much you love bacon and eggs, you're going to lust for a slice of toast and marmalade and a glass of orange juice to go with that breakfast. The accelerated weight loss is due to the lack of liquids. And tests have shown that, after no more than six months, most low-carb dietitians typically leave the system.

- Low-fat diets confuse dietitians— and prospective book readers— with the notion that you can consume all you like yet lose weight. Theoretically, it's valid since low-fat meals are typically fatty yet satisfying. But, like low-carb diets, these schemes quickly get very dull, mainly if they are vegetarian diets.

5.2 Preventive Snacking

Most people have done this "preventive snacking" without knowing it. Whoever cooks the dinner in the evening will always taste food while preparing. When peeling the carrots, most of us can eat one or two. Both my wife and I prefer to split the heel and enjoy it before starting on the bread. Do it a couple of days, and blood sugar starts to increase and then dinner is served to the rest of the family one isn't as hungry as well.

Consider snacking pre-emptive a part of your lifestyle. Start by getting breakfast. Sip your juice glass or have a slice of toast with twenty to thirty minutes of the first cup of coffee before settling down to the main meal. If you've "brown-bagged it" for lunch at work, you're not going to overeat because that bag can hold a small amount of food only even if you're going for lunch, mind getting the snack before leaving.

In the end, the dream will never be to get very hungry. Make sure you have one more balanced midafternoon snack. This is not about the usual doughnut and coffee. Instead, give it a pinch of dried fruit or almonds, or maybe a granola bar.

The evening meal presents the biggest temptation of overeating. Rather than waiting for dinner to be eaten, whether or not you are preparing it, get into the right routine of eating a reasonably small snack well before dinner. I enjoy all-grain crackers with some herring.

Or I might get a cup of yogurt. I hold precut vegetables bite-size— the French call these crudités — in the fridge to munch on while watching the nightly news as my wife cooks dinner or when I prepare dinner when it's my turn to eat.

For a couple of weeks, consider strategic snacking to see how it doesn't help you consume less at big meals. To be more productive, have a list of nutritious snacks on hand, and they're ready to be available.

5.3 Stop Stress Eating

I enjoy living in this new era with all its significant advantages and rewards, but for most of us, depression is a fact of life.

The higher the tension level during the day, the more likely we are to use eating as a calming strategy throughout the evening. We continuously eat, not because we are starving, but actually as a nervous impulse. I suppose it's a healthier habit than taking self-medication with booze during anesthesia, but it's also not safe.

The emphasis will be on the word habit in the last paragraph.

In the evening, we get into a profoundly ingrained habit of nonstop eating, particularly while watching TV or a DVD. There are a couple of options to deal with the bad habit.

The best thing to do is to accept the pattern, and then try to improve it a little. Speak to a snack in your evening. If you're like other men, you'll go to the freezer or pantry and grab the first food you'll find. If the meal turned out to be crispy potato chips, that's what you're going to eat, and you're going to devour the entire bag most definitely.

Rather than feeding yourself a little ice cream dish, you'll pull the bowl out and dive in with a spoon, even before the ice cream is finished.

Let's change those patterns. And if those chips are not in the pantry at all, so you find a few nuts in their shells instead? Place a couple or two along with a nutcracker in a tub and fish out the nutmeats in front of the TV. The idea is to keep your hands occupied shelling off the nuts instead of consuming mixed nuts from a pan.

Create your popcorn from scratch instead of cooking the varieties of microwaves that are filled with trans-fatty acids. The aromas that fill the house are exquisite and place you in a far more relaxed state.

The option I much prefer is to make a steaming cup of hot chocolate. High in fat and calories, this cup of cocoa relaxes the mind and, due to its polyphenol content, can help reduce blood pressure. For planning tips, see the recipe section at the end of the book. I consider that after drinking a cup of coffee, I get a much better night's sleep.

Keep one of those squeezable rubber balls or stress beads or something else nearby as a complete solution to snacking, to use your hands instead of eating. Try placing a few lightweight dumbbells next to the sofa or chair to start doing some exercise.

And seek to crack the cycle of conditioned-response entirely. Many of us are like Pavlov's dogs in a way, trained to eat as we sit in our current chair or couch, and the show continues. Read a novel, or journal, to break the habit. Don't turn the TV on either.

You'll need both hands to keep the book or journal, maybe to play some music. Because you are not used to snacking when blogging, you are not going to.

I have a specific house rule allowing zero food or alcohol in the bedroom. Thinking I'm tempted to eat, occasionally to excess, when I'm under tension and watching TV, or I'm tempted to go upstairs to the couch. I'll either do some reading or watching TV there, but I'm programmed not to eat in that room. Think of your own snacking and addiction, and work consciously to change certain behavioral habits.

5.4 Learning Portion Control

A guideline for healthy eating has been established in every country in the world. Most of us eat a wide range of foods per day to make sure you get all the nutrition you need.

Minimum five servings of fruit and vegetables will be the foundation of a balanced diet every day. I feel that, as many other authorities, if not most, are unified, the minimum should be up to nine servings a day. Second, these plant foods contain very few calories per meal. A meal is much smaller than the average consumer would consider.

A serving of fruit may be one medium apple, banana, pear, or peach, as described by nutritionists. Or, it may be two figs, 15 oranges, 2/3 cups of fruit, or half cups of applesauce.

If you eat dried fruit, just two teaspoons of raisins, two small plums, or four apple rings are consumed. Only 6 ounces of juice is a part of citrus. Start the day with a glass of milk and cold breakfast with a sliced banana, and a cup of fruit for two-thirds gives you three bat portions.

Pick a few raisins or prunes for a snack, and you are up to 4. Then maybe at dinner, you have sliced mango to a total of five servings of fruit for the day.

What's the matter with vegetables? Similarly, tiny volumes are a part. It's one cup of raw vegetables. A half-cup of tomato or other vegetable juice (4 ounces/120 ml) is a portion. A serving of cooked produce is just one-half cup (4 ounces).

Usually, a bowl of soup would have two portions of vegetables. What you probably will think will be one serving if you had planted on a plate actually would be two or, in restaurants, perhaps three.

The one thing that has shown up time and again in scientific trials without any contrary evidence is that people whose diets are high in fruit and vegetables have lower blood pressure and fewer heart problems and strokes, safe from cardiovascular disease.

The same applies to whole grain bread and cereals. Most food guides require three to four portions a day. Reduce the quantity of food in this segment made with refined flour, including pasta, white bread, cakes, and chocolate goods in terms of weight management. Please remember that a serving of cooked spaghetti is one cup of approximately 200 calories — not the big 3-cup piles you sometimes see.

Start talking about meats and food. A serving of any meat sort is around 3 1/2 ounces, around the size of a play card pack or of a man's hand. A steak of 1 pound is not one meal! A serving of some kind of cheese is 1 ounce. Consider a cheddar, a fontina, or a swiss1-inch square piece.

Only learning to judge weights and diet correctly would help you lose weight and keep losing weight.

Mind that it's a gradual change of habits, not just to lose weight in a couple of months.

5.5 Lose Excess Pounds and Watch Your Waistline.

Blood pressure is regularly rising as weight decreases. Getting overweight will also induce respiratory disorder when you are sleeping (sleep apnea), which raises blood pressure.

Weight reduction is one of the essential improvements in blood pressure management lifestyle. When you are overweight or obese, only a minimal amount of weight will help to reduce your blood pressure. Generally, for every kg (about 2.2 pounds) of weight, you lose, you can get your blood pressure by about 1 mm hg).

In addition to dumping pounds, you should usually keep an eye on your waistline. When you weigh so much around the hips, you will be more vulnerable to elevated blood pressure.

In total, people lose more than 40 inches (102 centimeters) of waist length.

Women are at risk if their estimation of waist reaches 35 inches (89 cm).

These numbers differ between ethnic groups. Tell the doctor for a proper assessment of your stomach.

5.6 Relieve Stress.

Persistent stress can raise blood pressure. Reduce stress. More work on the impact of chronic stress on blood pressure is needed. Occasional stress can also lead to high blood pressure when you respond to stress by consuming mediocre food, drinking, or smoking.

Take time to think about how busy you are, such as jobs, families, investments, or sickness. Once you know what causes stress, think about how you can reduce or eliminate stress.

If all the stressors cannot be removed, you can at least treat them more safely. Try to change your perceptions. Change your standards. Start your day and reflect on your goals, for example. Do not do too much, and learn to say no. Understand, you can't alter or control those events, so you should concentrate on adapting to them.

• You should concentrate on problems and prepare to fix them. Start talking to the boss if you have a question at work. When your child or partner is in dispute, take action to settle it.

• Stop stress-causing causes. Seek to prevent stimuli if necessary. For example, if rush-hour traffic creates frustration on the way to work, consider driving early in the morning or use public transport. If necessary, stop people that cause you pain.

• Take your time to rest and enjoy your hobbies. Take the time to relax and breathe slowly every day. You are taking time for fun sports or amusements, such as cycling, cooking, or volunteering.

• Express thankfulness. Thanksgiving to others can significantly relieve tension.

5.7 Other Blood Pressure Management Tips

Some other blood pressure reduction tips are discussed below:
1. Sleep rising sleep alone cannot cure high blood pressure, but too little sleep and bad quality of sleep will make it worse.

A 2015 review of Korean national health survey results found that people who sleep less than five hours a night suffer from hypertension more.

2. Per cigarette you smoke raises your blood pressure for several minutes after you are finished.

Stopping smoke tends to normalize blood pressure. Quitting smoking will reduce the chance of heart disease and improve your health overall. People who quit smoking will live longer than people who never stop smoking.

3. Cutting caffeine, the role of caffeine in blood pressure remains under debate. In people who rarely consume caffeine, blood pressure up to 10 mm hg can increase. Nevertheless, people who frequently drink coffee can have little to no effect on their blood pressure.

Despite the fact that the long-term effects of caffeine on blood pressure are not apparent, the blood pressure will rise significantly.

Test the pulse within 30 minutes of drinking a caffeinated coffee to see if caffeine raises the blood pressure. If your blood pressure rises by 5 to 10 mm hg, you might be prone to the influence of caffeine on your blood pressure. Speak to the doctor about the blood pressure effects of caffeine

4. Limit your alcohol consumption can be healthy as well as harmful for your health. You will lower your blood pressure by around 4 mm hg if you drink alcohol in excess — usually one drink a day for women or two a day for men. One cocktail is equal to 12 oz of beer, five ounces of champagne, or 1, 5 ounces of 80-solid liquor.

But if you drink too much alcohol, the preventive influence is lost.

Alcohol intake is higher than average levels will potentially increase blood pressure by many measures. This may also be high in the effectiveness of blood pressure medications.

5. Reduce sodium in your diet. If you have high blood pressure, only a modest reduction in the sodium in your intake will boost your heart health and reduce blood pressure by around 5 to 6 mm Hg.

The result of sodium intake on blood pressure differs between population groups. We are limiting sodium to 2,300 milligrams (mg) a day or less, in general. A lower intake of sodium— 1,500 mg a day or less— is, therefore, optimal for most adults.

Follow these tips to lower the sodium in your diet:

• Read food labels. Select low-sodium versions of the foods and beverages you usually purchase.

• Consume less of the packaged food. Just a small amount of sodium is naturally found in foods. Most sodium is applied as it is stored.

• Do not apply salt to them. Simply one salt teaspoon amount contains 2,300 mg of sodium. To add flavor to your meal, using herbs or spices.

• The facility in this. If you do not feel like you should immediately reduce the sodium in your diet dramatically, slowly cut back. The palate is set to adapt over time.

6. Home monitoring will help you keep tabs on your blood pressure, make sure your lifestyle adjustments are useful, and alert you and your doctor to possible health problems. Blood pressure monitoring systems are widely available and without a prescription. Speak to your doctor about housekeeping before you start.

Regular doctor visits are also crucial for managing blood pressure. When you have firm control of your blood pressure, check with your doctor how much you need to monitor it. Your doctor may recommend that you test it regularly, or less frequently. If you are making any adjustments to your medication or other procedures, your doctor may recommend that you monitor your blood pressure two weeks after changes in your care and one week before your next appointment.

7. Get support family and friends who love you will help improve your health. They could encourage you to take care of yourself, drive you to the doctor's office or embark with you on an exercise program to keep your blood pressure down.

If you find the help that you need outside your family and friends, consider joining a support group. This will place you in touch with people who can give you an emotional or morale boost and offer practical advice for coping with your illness.

Chapter 6: Healthy Recipes to Control Blood Pressure and Lose Weight

(Part 1)

6.1 Some Foods That Help Lower Blood Pressure

1. Leafy Greens

Potassium supports the kidneys by urinating to get rid of more sodium. It, in effect, reduces blood pressure.

Rich in potassium, leafy greens include: roman lettuce arugula kale turnip greens collard spinach beet greens Swiss chard canned vegetables have also added sodium. Yet frozen vegetables contain as many nutrients as fresh vegetables, and can be stored easily. For a good, sweet green juice, you can combine these vegetables with bananas and nut milk too.

2. Berries

Berries are rich in compounds called flavonoids, mainly the blueberries. One study showed these compounds could prevent hypertension and help lower blood pressure.

Add berries (strawberries, raspberries, and blueberries) to your diet. In the morning, you can put them on your granola or cereal, or carry frozen berries on hand for a fast, healthy dessert.

3. Red Beets

Beets are rich in nitric oxide and can help to open the blood vessels and lower blood pressure. Researchers have found that the nitrates in beetroot juice decreased blood pressure in just 24 hours for study participants.

You can use either juice your beets, or cook and eat the whole root. Beetroot is delicious for stir-fries and stews when roasted or added. They can also be baked in chips. Be cautious when handling beets— the juice will stain your clothes and hands.

4. Skim Milk

Skim milk and yogurt skim milk are excellent calcium sources, and low in fat. They are also essential components of a diet to reduce blood pressure. When you don't like milk, you can opt for yogurt too.

Women who eat five or more servings of yogurt a week reported a 20 percent decrease in their risk of developing high blood pressure, according to the American heart association.

Seek to add granola, almond slivers, and fruits into your yogurt for other beneficial heart health. Be sure to test for added sugar when buying yogurt. The lower the amount of sugar per serving, the better.

5. Oatmeal

Suits the bill to lower your blood pressure by a high-fiber, low-fat, and low-sodium route. Eating breakfast oatmeal is a perfect way to be warming up for the day.

Overnight oats are a common alternative for breakfasts. Soak 1/2 cup of almond milk and 1/2 cup of rolled oats in a pan to produce them. Stir it and add fruit, granola, and cinnamon in the morning to taste.

6. Bananas

It is easier to eat potassium-rich foods than to take supplements. Slice a banana over a potassium-rich addition into your cereal or oatmeal. You can also make one for a quick breakfast or snack, along with a boiled egg.

7. Lettuce, Mackerel, and Omega-3 Fish

These are some great sources of lean protein. Fatty fish (mackerel and salmon) are rich in omega-3 fatty acids that can lower blood pressure, lower inflammation, and lower triglycerides. Truite contains vitamin d, in addition to these sources of food. Foods seldom contain vitamin d, and this hormone-like vitamin has blood pressure reducing properties.

One advantage of fish preparation is that it is accessible to cook and flavor. Put a salmon fillet in parchment paper and season with herbs, lemon, and olive oil to try. Bake the fish over 12-15 minutes in a preheated oven at 450 ° f.

8. Unsalted Seeds

Are high in magnesium, potassium, and other minerals that are used to lower blood pressure. Enjoy 1/4 cup of sunflower, pumpkin, or squash seeds as a mealtime snack.

9. Ail and Herbs

One review trusted source states that by increasing the amount of nitric oxide in the body, garlic could help reduce hypertension. Nitric oxide helps to lower blood pressure by facilitating vasodilatation, or the expansion of arteries.

It can also help you cut down on your salt consumption by adding aromatic herbs and spices into your daily diet. Examples of herbs and spices that can be used include basil, cinnamon, thyme, rosemary, etc.

10. Dark Chocolate

A 2015 study showed a lower risk of cardiovascular disease (CVD) associated with consuming dark chocolate. The research indicates that dark chocolate may equate up to 100 grams per day with a lower risk of CVD.

Dark chocolate contains more than 60% of the solids in cocoa and has less sugar than normal chocolate. You can add dark chocolate to some yogurt, or eat it as a balanced dessert with fruits like strawberries, blueberries, or raspberries.

Find a large variety of dark chocolate on amazon.com.

11. Pistachios

Pistachios are the right way of lowering blood pressure by decreasing peripheral vascular resistance, or narrowing of the blood vessels, and heart rate? One trusted source report showed a diet of one serving of pistachios a day helps to lower blood pressure.

Pistachios can be integrated into your diet by adding to crusts, pesto sauces, and salads or by consuming them plain as a snack.

12. Olive Oil

An example of good fat is olive oil. It includes polyphenols, which are compounds that fight against inflammation and can help to reduce blood pressure.

As part of the dash diet, olive oil will help you reach your two to three daily servings of fat (see below for more on this diet). It's also a perfect alternative to dressing up canola oil, butter, or popular salads.

13. Pomegranates

Pomegranates are a nutritious fruit you can enjoy as a juice or as raw? One research concluded that drinking a cup of pomegranate juice for four weeks once a day tends to reduce blood pressure in the short run.

Grapefruit juice is excellent with a good meal. For store-bought drinks, be sure to test the sugar content as the added sugars will offset the health benefits.

(Part 2)
Delicious Recipes for Lowering Blood Pressure

A few of these recipes call for an egg substitute for reducing cholesterol wherever possible. These recipes were, however, tested in the kitchen, and they taste great! Cooking oil spray is also used for fat reduction.

With my flavor doctor seasoning, many of those recipes are delicious, an excellent way to simplify the cooking. When you see an asterisk (*) in the methods next to a spice or flavoring, replace one or more flavor doctor shakes for that spice— to your taste.

6.2 Appetizers

Pupusas Revueltas with Chicken

Yield: 12 servings

Ingredients

1 pound of ground chicken 1 tbsp of vegetable oil 1/2 small onion, finely diced one garlic clove, minced* 1 medium green pepper, seeded and minced one small tomato, finely chopped 1/2 tsp of salt 5 cups of instant corn flour (masa harina) 6 cups of water 1/2 pound of low-fat mozzarella cheese, grated

Recipe:

1. Sauté chicken in oil in a non-stick skillet over low heat until chicken turns white. Stir the chicken constantly to prevent it from sticking.

2. Add onion, garlic, green potatoes, and tomatoes. Cook until the mixture of chicken is cooked by. Remove the skillet from the stove and allow the mixture to cool in the fridge.

3. While cooling the chicken mixture, place the flour in a large mixing bowl and stir in enough water to make a tortilla-like dough.

4. Blend in the cheese when the chicken mixture has cooled.

5. Divide the dough into 24 slices. Roll the dough into small balls with hands, and flatten each ball into a circle 1/2 inch thick. Put a spoonful of the mixture of chicken in the middle of each dough circle and bring the edges to the center. Flap the dough ball again until it is 1/2 inch thick.

6. Cook the pupusas on each side in a hot iron skillet, until golden brown.

Serving size: 2 pupusas

Each serving provides:

Calories: 291 Total fat: 6,5 g saturated fat: 3 g monounsaturated fat: 2 g polyunsaturated fat: 1,5 g Cholesterol: 31 mg Sodium: 211 mg potassium: 339 mg Carbohydrates: 41 g Sugar: 7 g total fiber: 17 g Iron: 2 mg calcium: 149 mg vitamin a: 0 IU vitamin c: 8 mg vitamin d:0 µg magnesium: 79 mg nutrients

Spicy and Sweet Meatballs

Yield: 12 serving

Ingredients

1/4 cup onion, 1 pound of lean ground beef 1/3 cup of fine dried breadcrumbs 1/4 cup of fresh parsley, 1/8 tsp of nutmeg* 1/4 cup of liquid non-1 egg white, 1/2 cup cranberries, 2 tsp of finely chopped dry mustard* 1/8 tsp of cayenne pepper* 1/2 cup of grape jelly 1 tsp of lemon juice

Recipe

1. Coat a small saucepan with spray to cook; place over medium heat.

2. Stir in the onion and sauté until soft.

3. Combine the onion in a bowl with the next six ingredients. Shape into 36 1 inch meatballs. Place the meatballs on a spray-coated baking sheet (with sides) and bake for 18 minutes at 375 ° f.

4. Meanwhile, combine the cranberries and remaining ingredients into a small saucepan to prepare the sauce. Cook over medium heat until cooked thoroughly.

5. Place the meatballs in a serving bowl, then pour over the sauce. Serve with chopped dentures.

Serve size: 3 meatballs

Each Serving Provides:

Calories: 95 Total fat: 1.2 g saturated fat: 0.5 g monounsaturated fat: 0.7 g polyunsaturated fat: 0 g Cholesterol: 20 mg Sodium: 55 mg potassium: 156 mg carbohydrate: 12 g Sugar: 2 g fiber: 0.5 g magnesium: 11 mg calcium: 12 mg Protein: 9 g Iron: 1 mg vitamin a: 7 IU vitamin c: 2 mg vitamin d: 0 µg nut

Curtido Cabbage Salvador

Yield: 8 servings

Ingredients:

One medium head cabbage, chopped two small carrots, grated one small onion, sliced 1/2 tsp dried red pepper (optional) 1/2 tsp oregano* 1 tsp olive oil 1 tsp light salt 1 tsp brown sugar 1/4 cup vinegar 1/2 cup water

Recipe:

1. Blanch the cob for 1 minute with boiling water. Dismantle the water.

2. In a large bowl, place the cabbage and add the rubbed carrots, sliced onion, red pepper, oregano, olive oil, salt, brown sugar, vinegar, and water.

3. Place in fridge at least 2 hours before serving.

4. Serve with revueltas pupusas (p. 56).

Serving size: 1 cup

Each Serving Provides:

Total: calories: 37 total fat: 1 g saturated fat: 0 g polyunsaturated fat: 0.5 g Cholesterol: 0 mg Sodium: 293 mg potassium: 375 mg monounsaturated fat: 0.5 g carbohydrates: 6 g carbohydrates: < 1 g total fiber: 1.5 g magnesium: 10 mg calcium: 27 mg Protein: 1 g Iron: 0.5 mg vitamin a: 516 IU vitamin c: 14 mg vitamin d:0 µg

Mexican Pozole

Yield: 10 servings

Ingredients:

One tablespoon of olive oil, 2 pounds lean beef, cubed (see note) 1 large onion, chopped one clove of garlic, finely chopped* 1/4 tsp of light salt 1/8 tsp of black pepper* 1/4 cup cilantro* 1 can (15 oz) stewed tomatoes 2 oz of tomato paste (no added salt) 1 can (1 lb, 13 oz) hominy

Note: skinless, boneless chicken can be used instead of beef cubes.

Recipe:

1. Heat oil in a large pot then sautés beef.

2. Add the onion, garlic, salt, pepper, coriander, and sufficient water to cover the meat. Cover the pot over low heat and cook until the meat is tender.

3. Stir in tomatoes and paste tomatoes. Continue to cook for some 20 minutes.

4. Add hominy, and continue to cook for another 15 minutes over low heat, stirring occasionally. Add water if too thick for desired consistency.

Each Serving Provides:

Calories: 214 Total fat: 6 g monounsaturated fat: 2.5 g polyunsaturated fat: 0.5 g saturated fat: 3 g Cholesterol: 48 mg Sodium: 328 mg potassium: 420 mg Carbohydrates: 18 g Sugar: 4 g total fiber: 22 g Protein: 22 g magnesium: 30 mg calcium: 29 mg Iron: 6.5 mg vitamin a: 25 IU vitamin c: 4 mg vitamin d: 0.2 µg nutrition

Spicy Marinated Shrimp Bowl

Yield: 15 servings

Ingredients

5 pounds fresh large shrimp, peeled and deveined, add 1/2 cup olive oil, 1/2 cup white or red vinegar, 11/2 tsp lemon peel, 1/4 cup lemon juice 2 tsp tomato paste (no salt added) 3 garlic cloves, 1/2 tsp light salt 1/4 tsp cayenne pepper* 1/2 tsp black pepper* 1/2 tsp white pepper, ground*

Recipe:

1. In the big pot, bring 5 quarts of water to a boil in a large kettle and then add shrimp. Remove to a boil, then reduce heat to a simmer. Simmer for 1 to 3 minutes, uncovered, or until shrimp is done. Shrimp drain. Rinse under running cold water; drain again.

2. For marinade, combine oil, vinegar, lemon peel, lemon juice, tomato paste, garlic, salt, and all three types of pepper into a screw-top jar.

Cover, and well shaken. Pour over the shrimp to marinade – cover overnight and chill.

Each serving provides:

Calories: 207 Total fat: 8.5 g monounsaturated fat: 5.5 g polyunsaturated fat: 1.5 g Cholesterol: 229 mg Sodium: 265 mg potassium: 369 mg carbohydrate: 2.5 g Sugar: 0 g total fiber: 0 g Iron: 3.8 mg magnesium: 58 mg calcium: 82 mg Protein: 30 g vitamin a: 88 IU vitamin c: 6 mg vitamin d: 5.5 µg nutrition: 82 mg vitamin a: 88

Black-Eyed Pea Salsa

Yield: 4 servings

Ingredients

1 can (15 oz) black-peas, rinsed and drained 1/4 cup thinly sliced green onion 1/4 cup red sweet pepper, chopped 2 tbsp of canola oil 2 tbsp of cider vinegar 1 to 2 fresh jalapeño peppers, seeded and chopped 1/4 tsp of black pepper* 2 cloves of garlic, minced*

Recipe:

1. Combine all the ingredients overnight in a pot, cover, and cool.

Serve size: 1/2 cup

Each Serving Provides:

Calories: 169 Total fat: 6.5 g saturated fat: 0.5 g monounsaturated fat: 4 g polyunsaturated fat: 2 g Cholesterol: 0 mg Sodium: 147 mg potassium: 507 mg carbohydrate: 24 g sugar:0 g dietary fiber: 5 g magnesium: 61 mg calcium: 146 mg Protein: 3.5 g Iron: 1.6 mg vitamin a: 135 IU vitamin c: 22 mg vitamin d: 0 µg nutrition

Pan-Fried Yucca

Yield: 6 servings

Ingredients:

1 pound of fresh yucca (cassava, sliced into 3-inch pieces and peeled)

Recipe:

1. Combine the yucca in a kettle with enough cold water to cover it by 1 inch. Bring the water at boiling level, and simmer the yucca for 20 to 30 minutes, or until tender.

2. Preheat oven to 350 degrees f.

3. Move the yucca to a cutting board with a slotted spoon, allow it to cool and cut lengthwise into 3/4-inch long wedges, discarding the thin woody center.

4. Spray cookie sheet with spray to cook. Place the yucca wedges on the baking sheet, and brush the cooking wedges with oil. Cover with paper foil and bake for eight minutes. Uncover and return to the oven for another 7 minutes to cook.

Serving size: 1 piece (21/2 inches long)

Each serving provides:

Calories: 116 Total fat: < 1 g saturated fat: < 1 g monounsaturated fat: 0 g polyunsaturated fat: 0 g Cholesterol: 0 mg Sodium: 3 mg potassium: 205 mg Carbohydrates: 28 g carbohydrates: 5 g total fiber: 1 g magnesium: 15 mg calcium: 66 mg Protein: 1 g Iron: 3 mg vitamin a: 1.5 IU vitamin c: 15.5 mg vitamin c: 1 g

Roasted Red Chili Pepper

Yield: 6 servings

Ingredients

1 can (16 oz) chickpeas or garbanzo beans 11/2 tsp cumin* 1 tsp coriander 1/4 tsp cayenne pepper* 1/2 tsp light salt 2 tbsp tahini 1 tbsp lemon juice 2 to 3 cloves garlic, pressed or crushed* 1/2 cup roasted red pepper fresh ground pepper to taste*

Recipe:

1. Drain and rinse the chickpeas/garbanzos, conserve the liquid.

2. Combine cumin, cilantro, cayenne, and salt in a small cup. Mix carefully.

3. Put chickpeas in the food processor bowl with chopping blade and sprinkle uniformly over the top of the spice mixture.

4. Add the tahini, lemon juice, garlic, and red pepper, then blend until well combined. Stir in the fresh ground pepper.

5. Once the hummus is smooth, add some liquid from the chickpeas while it is being processed until it reaches the desired consistency.

6. Serve with toasted pita bread, or with almost anything as a dip or spread.

Each serving contains:

Calories: 156 Total fat: 4 g saturated fat: 0.5 g monounsaturated fat: 1.5 g polyunsaturated fat: 2 g Cholesterol: 0 mg Sodium: 103 mg potassium: 394 mg carbohydrate: 23 g total fiber: 6 g Protein: 7 g Iron: 2.5 mg magnesium: 55 mg calcium: 47 mg sugar: 4 g vitamin a: 41 IU vitamin c: 14 mg vitamin d: 0 µg nutrition

Gazpacho

Yield: 4 servings Ingredients 3 medium tomatoes, peeled and chopped 1/2 cup cucumber, seeded and chopped 1/2 cup green pepper, chopped two green onions, sliced 2 cups low sodium vegetable juice cocktail 1 tbsp lemon juice 1/2 tsp basil, dried* 1/4 tsp hot pepper sauce* 1 clove garlic, hazelnut*

Recipe:

1. Combine all ingredients into a large mixing bowl.

2. Cover and freeze over for several hours in the refrigerator.

Every Serving Provides:

Calories: 65 Total fat: 1 g saturated fat: 0,5 g monounsaturated fat: 0,5 g Cholesterol: 0 mg Sodium: 41 mg potassium: 514 mg carbohydrate: 12 g total fiber: 2 g Protein: 2 g Iron: 1 mg magnesium: 15 mg calcium: 47 mg sugar: 1 g vitamin a: 178 IU vitamin c: 62 mg vitamin d:0 μg nutrition

Pesto Pita Bites

Yield: 4 servings

Ingredients

1 cup of fresh basil leaves* 2 garlic cloves* 2 to 3 tbsp parmesan cheese 1/4 cup olive oil one whole pita bread

Recipe:

1. Place the basil leaves until well chopped in a food processor. Attach the parmesan cheese with the garlic and 1 1/2 tablespoons and combine while gradually adding olive oil.

2. Divide the pita bread into two rings. Remove pesto mixture and sprinkle with cheese.

3. Cut each of them into six wedges, then each one of them on an ungreased baking sheet.

4. Bake for 10 to 12 minutes at 350of or until it is crisp. Serving hot.

Every Serving Provides:

Calories: 228 Total fat: 14 g saturated fat: 2.5 g monounsaturated fat: 10 g polyunsaturated fat: 1.5 g Cholesterol: 2.5 g Sodium: 150 mg potassium: 654 mg Carbohydrates: 20 g Sugar: 6 g dietary fiber: 8.5 g Iron: 9 mg magnesium: 89 mg calcium: 428 mg Protein: 5.5 g vitamin a: 174 IU vitamin c: 11.5 mg vitamin d:0 μg nutrition

Artichoke dip

Amount of servings

Serves 8

Ingredients

1 can (15.5 ounces) artichoke hearts in water, drained 4 cups of chopped raw spinach two cloves of garlic, minced one teaspoon of ground black pepper one teaspoon of minced fresh thyme (or 1/3 teaspoon of dried) 1 tablespoon of fresh minced parsley (or one teaspoon of dried)

Directions

In a mixing bowl, combine the ingredients. Switch to an oven-safe glass or ceramic dish and bake at 350 ft for 30 minutes. Serve yourself dry.

Nutritional analysis per serving

Serving size: around 1/2 cup Total carbohydrate10 g Dietary fiber6 g Sodium130 mg Saturated fat1 g Total fat2 g Trans fat0 g Cholesterol6 mg Protein5 g Unsaturated fat TraceCalories78 Added sugars0 g Total sugars1.5 g

Grilled pineapple

Dietitian tip:

This Caribbean-style marinade and grill heat provide this pineapple.

Amount of servings

Serves 8

Ingredients For marinade

two tablespoons of dark honey, one tablespoon of olive oil, one tablespoon of fresh lime juice, one teaspoon of ground cinnamon, 1/4 teaspoon of ground cloves, one healthy ripe pineapple, eight wooden skewers soaked in water for 30 minutes or metal skewers, one tablespoon of dark rum (optional), one tablespoon of grated lime.

Directions

1. Away from the heat source, gently brush the grill rack or grill pan with a cooking spray. Place the cooking rack 4 to 6 inches away from the heat source.
2. For a small cup, add the sugar, olive oil, lime juice, cinnamon, and cloves and the whisk to make the marinade. Place it aside.
3. Cut the crown off the leaves and the base of the pineapple. Stand the pineapple upright and, using a big, sharp knife, close the skin, cut it down just below the surface in thin, vertical strips, leaving the little brown "heads" on the fruit. Place the pineapple on its side. To align the knife blade with the diagonal rows of eyes, cut a shallow furrow, using a spiral pattern around the pineapple, to eliminate both eyes. Stand straight and cut the peeled pineapple in half lengthwise. Place through pineapple half of the cut-side down and cut it lengthwise into four long wedges; cut the core away. Split the crosswise wedge into three bits. Thread the three pieces of pineapple on each skewer.
4. Brush the pineapple with the marinade gently. Barbecue or barbecue, mixing once or twice with the remaining marinade, until tender and golden, about 5 minutes on each side.
5. Clear the pineapple from the skewers and place it on a tray or individual serving plates. Clean the rum, if it is used, and sprinkle with the lime zest. Serve hot or sweet.

Nutritional review per serving

Serving size: 1/8 pineapple and marinade Total carbohydrate 13g Dietary fiber 1g Sodium 1 mg Saturated fat<1 g Total fat 2 g Cholesterol 0 mg Protein <1 g Unsaturated fat 1g Calories 70 Added sugars 0g Trans-fat 0g

Parmesan Yogurt Dip

Ingredients

1 cup fat-free plain yogurt 1/4 cup grated parmesan cheese 1/4 cup reduced-fat sour cream three tablespoons minced fresh parsley one green onion, thinly sliced one teaspoon prepared mustard one teaspoon of onion powder 1/4 teaspoon salt 1/8 teaspoon of pepper added vegetables

Instructions

1. In a bowl, add yogurt, parmesan cheese, sour cream, parsley, green onion cover, and refrigerate for at least two hours. Serve with a variety of vegetables.

Nutrition facts

2 tablespoons: 30 calories, 1 g fat (1 g saturated fat), 4 mg cholesterol, 120 mg sodium, 3 g carbohydrate (0 sugar, 0 fiber), 2 g protein. Diabetic exchange: 1/2 starch.

Pork Medallions with Balsamic-Honey Glaze

Level: simple total: 20 min Prep: 8 min Cook: 12 min yield: 4 to 6 servings

Ingredients

4 cloves of garlic, finely chopped one tablespoon of fresh rosemary, plus rosemary branches for garnishing 1/2 cup balsamic vinegar three tablespoons of honey two tablespoons of olive oil one tablespoons Dijon mustard salt and freshly ground black.

Instructions

1. Put the garlic and the rosemary in a small cup. Add the vinegar, sugar, olive oil, mustard, salt, and pepper to taste and stir to mix.
2. Slice the tenderloin into 1-inch thick medallions (rounds). Cover the bottom of the medium skillet with a light canola oil film and run over medium-longing run until dry. Attach the pork slices in 1 plate, season with salt and pepper, and simmer for 1 minute. Turn and sauté for

another 1 minute until lightly browned. Move the slices to a shallow baking dish in 1 layer.
3. Pour the glass over the slices and transfer to the cover.
4. Roast for 8 to 10 minutes, until the inserted thermometer hits 140 degrees f for medium. Remove from the oven and keep warm and loosely covered until ready to eat.
5. Place pork medallions on a plate and spoon the balsamic-honey glaze over them. Garnish with the rosemary sprigs on the pan.

6.3 Beverages

Blackberry iced tea with cinnamon and ginger

Dietitian tip: most herbal teas are free of caffeine.

Amount of servings

Serves 6

Ingredients

Six cups water 12 blackberry herbal tea bags eight 3-inch-long cinnamon sticks one tablespoon minced fresh ginger 1 cup unsweetened cranberry juice Sugar substitute to taste Ice cubes, crushed

Instructions

1. In a large saucepan, heat water just before boiling. Remove tea bags, two cinnamon sticks, and ginger. Remove from oil, cover, and let it steep for about 15 minutes.
2. Pass the mixture through a fine-mesh sieve, which is placed over a pitcher. To try, apply the juice and the sweetener. Refrigerate until very cold.
3. To serve, fill six large glasses with crushed ice. Pour the tea over the ice cubes and garnish with cinnamon sticks. Serve right now.

Nutritional analysis per serving

Serving size: 1 cup plus ice Total carbohydrate6 g Dietary fiber trace Sodium3 mg Saturated fat0 g Total fat0 g Trans fat0 g Cholesterol0 mg Protein Trace Unsaturated fat0 g Calories25 Added sugars0 g Total sugars5 g

Blueberry lavender lemonade

Dietitian tip: for better performance, carefully weigh lavender and buy fresh lemon juice— not concentrate — or squeeze around ten big lemons.

Amount of servings

Serves 16

Ingredients

2 cups water one pack (16 ounces) blueberries 1/4 cup granulated sugar one tablespoon dried lavender flowers 1 cup lemon juice two tablespoons Splenda sweetener Coldwater

Instructions

1. In a 1-gallon bowl, add 4 cups of ice and set aside. Bring 2 cups of water to a boil in a medium saucepan. In the pan, add the blueberries, sugar, and lavender. Boil for about 5 minutes, until the blueberries have popped and all the sugar has dissolved.
2. Strain the mixture of blueberry over the pitcher of ice; discard the remaining blend of blueberry. Apply the juice of the lemon and the Splenda to the cup. Fill the top with cold water. Mix well, guy.

Nutritional review per serving

Serving size: 8 ounces Calories33 Total fat0 g Saturated fat0 g Trans fat0 g Unsaturated fat0 g Cholesterol0 mg Sodium7 mg Total carbohydrate8 g Dietary fiber0 g Total sugars7 g Protein0 g

Cranberry spritzer

Dietitian tip: to reduce calories, even more, using a low-calorie sweetener instead of sugar.

Amount of servings

Serves 10

Ingredients

1-quart reduced-calorie cranberry juice 1/2 cup fresh lemon juice 1-quart saltwater 1/4 cup sugar 1 cup raspberry sherbet ten lemon or lime wedges

Instructions

1. Refrigerate cranberry juice, lemon juice, and carbonated water until cooled.
2. In a big pitcher, mix cranberry juice, lemon juice, carbonated soda, sugar, and sherbet. Pour in small chilled glasses and garnish with lemon or lime wedges. Serve right now.

Nutritional analysis per serving

Serving size: 1 cup Total fat trace Calories100 Protein Trace Cholesterol0 mg Total carbohydrate24 g Dietary fiber trace unsaturated fat Trace Saturated fat Trace Trans fat0 g Sodium9 mg Addedsugars10 g Total sugars22 g

Fresh fruit smoothie

Dietitian's tip: you can prepare ingredients in advance and place them in the refrigerator until you're ready to mix.

Amount of servings

Serves 4

Ingredients

one cup fresh pineapple chunks, 1/2 cup cantaloupe or other melon chunks, 1 cup fresh strawberries Juice, two oranges, 1 cup cold water, one tablespoon honey

Instructions

1. Extract pineapple and melon rind. Cut the pieces. Cut the strawberry stems. Place all ingredients in a blender and purée until smooth. Serve in the rain.

Nutritional overview per serving

Serving size: 8 ounces Total carbohydrate17 g Dietary fiber1 g Sodium7 mg Saturated fat0 g Total fat0 g Trans fat0 g Cholesterol0 mg Protein1 g Unsaturated fat0 g Calories72 Added sugars4 g Natural sugars13 g

High-protein smoothie

Dietitian tip: add one tablespoon of linseed oil for an extra 120 calories, 14 grams of fat, and no added sodium or cholesterol to make the recipe higher in calories.

Amount of servings

Serves 1

Ingredients

One cup vanilla yogurt 1 cup 2 percent milk, one medium banana, two tablespoons wheat germ two tablespoons protein powder

Instructions

1. In a blender, mix yogurt, milk, banana chunks, wheat germ, and protein powder. Mix until it's smooth. Pour into a durable chilled bottle and serve it immediately.

Nutritional analysis per serving

Serving size: 2 and half to 3 cups Calories 608 Total fat 20 g Saturated fat 9 g Trans-fat 0.2 g Unsaturated fat 4 g Cholesterol 57 mg Sodium 301 mg Total carbohydrate 75 g Dietary fiber 7 g Total sugar 53 g Added sugars 4 g Protein 32 g

Healthy expresso

Dietitian's tip: Espresso is an excellent dark coffee that is also the basis for other beverages. The iced version contains brown sugar and almond syrup. You can use some additional flavored syrup, such as hazelnuts, or you can skip the flavoring.

Number of servings

Serves 4

Ingredients

2 cups of decaffeinated espresso coffee, two tablespoons of golden brown sugar 1 1/2 cups of fat-free milk two tablespoons of sugar-free almond syrup* Ice cubes 1 cup of fat-free whipped topping* 1 teaspoon of ground espresso beans* Note: If you need to follow a gluten-free diet, check the labels to be sure the brands of syrup and

Instructions

1. In a bowl, add espresso, brown sugar, milk, and syrup. Stir to balance it uniformly. Refrigerate until cold.
2. Fill out four glasses of ice cubes. Pour some coffee over the ice. Attach 1/4 cup of whipped topping to each drink and sprinkle with ground espresso beans.

Nutritional analysis per serving

Serving size: 1 glass (about eight fluid ounces) Cholesterol 3 mg Calories 70 Sodium 69 mg Total fat 1 g Total carbohydrate 11 g Saturated fat 1 g Dietary fiber 0 g Total fat 0 g Added sugars 7 g Unsaturated fat Trace Protein 4 g.

Non-alcoholic margarita

Dietitian's tip: this recipe makes a more uncomplicated syrup than you'll need. Hold the excess in the refrigerator for a few days.

Amount of servings

Serves 2

Ingredients Simple syrup:

1/2 cup sugar 1/2 cup water Margaritas: 2 cups ice 1/2 cup fresh lime juice three tablespoons simple syrup Cut fresh fruit to garnish

Instructions

1. In a small saucepan, heat sugar and water. Stir until the sugar has dissolved. Remove from heat and refrigerate.
2. Apply ice, juice, and natural syrup to the blender. Mix until smooth, pour in the desired chilled glass, and garnish the rim with the cut fruit.

Nutritional review per serving

Serving size: 8 ounces Total carbohydrate 17 g Dietary fiber trace Sodium 2 mg Saturated fat 0 g Total fat 0 g Trans-fat 0 g Cholesterol 0 mg Protein Trace Unsaturated fat 0 g Calories 68 Added sugars 12 g Total sugars 13 g

Strawberry mockarita

Dietitian's tip: this non-alcoholic drink is a festive way to start or finish your meal.

Amount of servings

Serves 6

Ingredients

Four cups of chopped strawberries 1/4 cup lime juice 1/4 cup sugar 2 cups water 2 cups ice

Instructions

1. Put all parts in a blender. Mix until it's smooth.

Nutritional review per serving size:

8 ounces Calories64 Total fat0 g Saturated fat0 g Trans fat0 g Unsaturated fat0 g Cholesterol0 mg Sodium3 mg Total carbohydrate16 g Dietary fiber2 g Total sugars13 g Protein1 g

Yogurt Breakfast Drink

Ingredients

2 cups of vanilla yogurt 2 cups of peach yogurt 1/2 cup of thawed orange juice concentrate 1/2 cup of fat-free milk 2 cups of ice cubes

Instructions

1. In a blender, mix the first four ingredients; cover and process until smooth. Attach the ice cubes, cover, and cycle until smooth. Pour in glasses; serve immediately.

Health Facts

1 cup: 166 calories, 2 g fat (1 g saturated fat), 10 mg cholesterol, 100 mg sodium, 30 g carbohydrate (0 sugar, 0 fiber), 8 g protein. Diabetic exchange: 1 apple, one fat-free milk.

Dark Chocolate Avocado Mousse

Servings: 4 (1/2 cup each)

Ingredients

2 small ripe avocados 1/4 cup non-sweetened cocoa powder 1/4 cup honey 1/4 cup dark chocolate chips or minced dark chocolate 1/2 cup milk of choice 1/2 teaspoon vanilla

Preparation

1. Cut avocados in half and cut seeds. Scoop from shells to a blender or a food processor.

2. Place chocolate chips in a microwave-safe container and heat in 30 seconds, stirring until smooth.
3. Attach the melted chocolate and remaining ingredients to the blender and combine until smooth. Divide in 4 serving dishes and refrigerate at least one hour before serving.

Ingredient Combinations and Substitutions

Egg-free and vegetable-free egg of choice and sugar-free chocolate chips are used. I am using maple syrup or agave instead of honey for vegan.

Cooking and Serving Tips

Apply more milk to the teaspoon, if necessary, until the desired consistency is achieved.

Extra-Dark Honey Sweetened Hot Cocoa

Servings: 2 (6-ounce cup each)

Ingredients

1 1/2 cup skim milk (or milk of choice) 1 1/2 tablespoons honey two tablespoons of unsweetened dark chocolate cocoa powder 1/4 tsp vanilla extract marshmallows for coating (optional)

Preparation

1. In a medium saucepan, heat over medium-low heat and whisk until cocoa has dissolved.
2. Remove the remaining milk and continue to heat until simmering.
3. Remove from heat and whisk in the vanilla mixture. If you like, pour in two mugs and top with marshmallows.

Ingredient Combinations and Substitutions

For the milk-free version, using a plant-based option such as almond or soy milk.

Using plant-based milk and substitute honey for maple syrup for vegan cocoa.

You are using the highest quality cocoa powder that you can find for the best results.

Cooking and serving tips turn on low heat to prevent scorching or curdling milk.

Heat cups in advance to keep the cocoa heat after serving.

Food Highlights (Per Serving)

124 calories 1 g fat 25 g carbs 7 g protein

Strawberry-Banana Soy Smoothie

Ingredients

2 cups of fresh strawberries, stemmed and halved (about ten berries) $1 1/2 cups of vanilla low-fat soy milk 1 1/2 teaspoons of honey 1/2 teaspoon of vanilla extract one banana, sliced 1 cup of frozen fat-free whipped topping, thawed

Preparation:

1. In a blender, add the first five ingredients of the recipe; process until smooth. Cover each serving with 1/4 cup of whipped topping. Serve right away.

6.4 Breads

Hawaiian Bread

12 servings per loaf

Ingredients

1/3 cup sugar 1/3 cup margarine 1/2 cup egg substitute 2 cup flour 3 tsp baking powder 1 cup crushed pineapple (in its juice), drained six maraschino cherries, minced

Recipe:

1. Beat the margarine and sugar until soft and fluffy.

2. Remove the egg substitute and blend well.

3. In a separate dish, combine the flour and baking powder. Combine mixtures of the sugar and flour. Mix. Blend.

4. Stir in pineapple and cherries and blend. Pour into 9-5-inch greased pan.

5. Bake for 1 hour, at 350 ° f.

Each Serving Provides:

Calories: 136 Total fat: 2 g monounsaturated fat: 0.5 g saturated fat: 0.5 g cholesterol: < 1 mg sodium: 51 mg potassium: 87 mg carbohydrate: 26 g Sugar: 10 g dietary fiber: 1 g magnesium: 8.5 mg calcium: 12 mg Iron: 1.2 mg vitamin c: 2 mg vitamin d: < 1 µg vitamin a: 47.8 iu nutrition

Zucchini Bread

yield: 16 servings per loaf

Ingredients

3/4 cup egg substitute 1 1/2 cups of sugar 1 cup of applesauce 2 cups of unpeeled zucchini, 1 tsp of vanilla 2 cups of flour 1/4 tsp of baking powder 1 tsp of baking soda, add 1 tsp of cinnamon, 1/2 tsp of ginger 1 cup of unpeeled nuts

Recipe

1. Match egg substitution.

2. In the eggs, add sugar, applesauce, zucchini, and vanilla.

3. Sift dry ingredients together in a separate pot and add to the mixture.

4. Pour into a loaf saucepan and bake for 1 hour at 375 ° f.

5. Cut 16 strips.

Every Serving Provides:

Calories: 200 Total fat: 4.5 g saturated fat: 0.5 g monounsaturated fat: 1 g polyunsaturated fat: 3 g cholesterol: < 1 mg sodium: 108 mg potassium: 118 mg carbohydrate: 35 g Sugar: 12 g total fiber: 1.5 g Iron: 1.3 mg magnesium: 21.5 mg calcium: 20 mg Protein: 5 g Sugar: 6 g vitamin a: 29 IU vitamin c: 1.4 mg vitamin d: < 1 µg nutrition

Raspberry Streusel Muffins

Yield: 16 muffins

Ingredients

1 1/3 cup flour 1 1/2 tsp baking powder 1 cup fresh or frozen raspberries 1/4 cup margarine 1/4 cup sugar 1/4 cup egg substitute 1/2 cup liquid non-dairy creamer 1/4 cup brown sugar 1/4 cup flour 2 tsp margarine 2 tsp cinnamon

Recipe:

1. Preheat to 375 ° f in the oven. Label 16 paper liner muffin cups.

2. Mix 1 1/3 cups of flour and baking powder in a medium pot. Stir the raspberries.

3. In a separate dish, mix 1/4 cup of margarine with sugar and egg substitute. Blend the creamer.

4. Stir in flour mixture until it has just been moistened. Spoon to 16 cups of muffin.

5. In a small bowl, mix brown sugar, 1/4 cup flour, two teaspoons margarine, and cinnamon. Sprinkle with muffins and cook for about 15 minutes.

Serving size: 1 muffin

Per Serving Contains:

Calories: 118 Total fat: 2 g saturated fat: 0.5 g unsaturated fat: 0.5 g polyunsaturated fat: 1 g cholesterol: < 1 mg sodium: 81 mg potassium: 53 mg Carbohydrates: 23 g Sugar: 6 g dietary fiber: 1 g Protein: 1.8 g Iron: 1 mg magnesium: 5.5 mg calcium: 37 mg vitamin a: 28.5 IU vitamin c: 2 mg vitamin d: < 1 μg

Zucchini Bread

Yield: 16 servings per loaf

Ingredients

3/4 cup egg substitute 1 1/2 cup sugar 1 cup apple sauce 2 cups unpeeled zucchini, 1 tsp vanilla 2 cups flour 1/4 tsp baking powder 1 tsp soda 1 tsp cinnamon 1/2 tsp ginger 1 cup unpeeled, chopped nuts

Recipe:

1. Beat the egg substitute.

2. Mix the butter, apple sauce, courgettes, and vanilla into the eggs.

3. Put the dry ingredients together in a different bowl and add them to the mixture.

4. Pour in the loaf pan and bake at 375 ° f for 1 hour.

5. Split the mixture into 16 slices.

Each Serving Provides:

Calories: 200 Total fat: 4.5 g saturated fat: 0.5 g unsaturated fat: 1 g polyunsaturated fat: 3 g cholesterol: < 1 mg sodium: 108 mg potassium: 118 mg Carbohydrates: 35 g Sugar: 12 g dietary fiber: 1.5 g Protein: 5 g Iron: 1.3 mg magnesium: 21.5 mg calcium: 20 mg vitamin a: 29 IU vitamin c: 1.4 mg vitamin d: < 1 μg nutrition

Whole Wheat Pop-Overs

Yield: 12 servings

Ingredients

1 1/4 cups all-purpose flour 3/4 cup whole wheat flour 3/4 tsp salt 2 cups low-fat milk 1 cup egg substitute 2 tbsp melted butter, refrigerated

Recipe:

1. Preheat the oven to a temperature of 450 ° f.

2. In a medium dish, mix flour and salt.

3. In a separate bowl, mix milk, egg substitute and butter with a low-speed blender. Connect the dry ingredients slowly and process until smooth.

4. Spray two 12 cup muffin pans with a cooking spray; pour in the batter, filling each with around 3/4 of the mixture — bake for 15 minutes.

5. Decrease the oven temperature to almost 350 ° f and bake for another 15 to 20 minutes.

Serving size: 2 popovers

Per Serving Contains:

Calories: 107 total fat: 3 g saturated fat: 1.5 g unsaturated fat: 1 g polyunsaturated fat: 0.5 g cholesterol: 7 mg sodium: 151 mg potassium: 275 mg carbohydrates: 17 g sugar: 5 g dietary fiber: 1.3 g protein: 3 g iron: 1 mg magnesium: 20 mg calcium: 66 mg vitamin a: 87 iu vitamin c: 0.5 mg vitamin d: 0.6 µg.

Blueberry Oat Bran Muffins

Yield: 12 muffins

Ingredients

1 1/2 cups of oat bran 1 1/8 cups of apple sauce 1 1/2 cups of all-purpose flour 1/2 cup of egg substitute 1/2 cup of brown sugar 2 tsp of canola oil 2 tsp of soda 1 tsp of vanilla extract 2 tsp of baking powder 1 1/2 cups of blueberries 1 tsp of ground cinnamon 1/4 ounce of sliced pecans 1/2 tsp of salt 1/2 cup of low-fat granola

Recipe:

1. Preheat oven to 400 degrees f. Line a 12-cup muffin pan with paper muffin liners, then spray the cooking spray liners.

2. Put and mix the oat bran, flour, brown sugar, baking soda, baking powder, cinnamon, and salt in a big bowl.

3. Blend the egg substitute, canola oil, applesauce, and vanilla extract in a separate pot. Mix the applesauce blend entirely into the flour mixture.

4. Throw the pecans and blueberries back. Spoon the whole batter into the cups of the prepared muffins. Sprinkle the granola batter, then gently force the granola to adhere.

5. Bake in the preheated oven for 18 minutes or clean until a toothpick inserted into a muffin comes out. Excellent, on a rack of wire.

Serving size: 1 muffin

Each Serving Provides:

Calories: 218 Total fat: 4 g monounsaturated fat: 2 g polyunsaturated fat: 1.5 g saturated fat: 0.5 g cholesterol: < 1 mg sodium: 260 mg Carbohydrates: 40 g Sugar: 15 g total fiber: 3.5 g Protein: 5.5 g Iron: 2 mg magnesium: 40 mg calcium: 72 mg potassium: 260 mg vitamin a: 43 IU vitamin c: 2.8 mg vitamin d: < 1 µg protein: 5.5 g Iron: 2 mg

Oatmeal Bread

Yield: 2 loaves

Ingredients

4 cups of all-purpose flour plus 1 pack of active dry yeast 1/4 cup of water 1/3 cup of brown sugar 3 tbsp of margarine 1 tsp of salt 1/2 tsp of cinnamon 2 cups of rolled oats

Recipe:

1. Combine 2 cups of all-purpose flour and leaven in a large mixing bowl; set aside.

2. Heat and mix water, brown sugar, margarine, salt, and cinnamon in a medium saucepan until it is warm, and the margarine almost melts. Add the liquid mixture to a mixture of flour/yeast.

3. Beat for 30 seconds with an electric mixer on low to medium speed. Then, beat for 3 minutes on high. Then stir in the dried oats and all-purpose flour left over.

4. Knead in all-purpose flour to make a moderately steep dough which is smooth and elastic on a lightly floured surface.

Shape the dough into a ball. Place the dough in a slightly grated bowl; transform to grease surface once. Cover and let the dough rise until double in size (1 to 1 1/2 hours) at a warm spot.

5. When the dough has doubled in thickness, force down your fist into the dough center. Turn onto a gently floured surface then split in half.

6. Form each dough by patting or rolling, half into a loaf.

7. Place halves of dough in 2 lightly greased loaf pans. Cover and let it grow again in a sunny position until almost double in size (~35-40 minutes).

8. Preheat oven to 375 degrees f. Bake 35-40 minutes. (For the last 10 minutes, bread can need to be loosely covered with foil to avoid over-browning.) Immediately remove food from the loaf pans and cool on wire rack.

Serving size: 12 portions per loaf

Each Serving Provides:

Calories: 103 Total fat: 1 g saturated fat: < 1 g monounsaturated fat: < 1 g polyunsaturated fat: 0.5 g Cholesterol: 0 mg Sodium: 60 mg potassium: 115 mg Carbohydrates: 21 g Sugar: 11 g dietary fiber: 2.5 g magnesium: 10.5 mg calcium: 8 mg Iron: 1 mg vitamin a: 6.74 IU vitamin c: 0 mg vitamin d vitamin c:

English Muffin Bread

Yield: 2 loaves

Ingredients

6 cups of all-purpose flour two packs of active dry yeast 1/4 cup of baking soda 2 cups of low-fat milk 1/2 cup of water 1 cup of sugar 1 cup of salt 3/4 cup of cornmeal

Recipe:

1. Grease 2 loaf pans and sprinkles thinly on greased pans with cornmeal to cover the bottoms and sides. Put away plates.

2. Combine 1/2 of the flour, yeast, and baking soda into a large mixing bowl; set aside.

3. Heat and mix milk, water, sugar, and salt until moist, in a medium saucepan. Then stir in the milk mixture and add in the remaining flour.

4. In prepared loaf pans, divide the dough in half and put it. Sprinkle cornmeal over the edges. In a warm spot, cover and let rise until double in size (~45 minutes).

5. Preheat oven to 400 degrees f. Bake for 25 minutes or until cooked in golden color. Lift immediately from pans and cool on rack wire.

Serving size: 12 portions per loaf

Each Serving Provides:

Calories: 135 Total fat: 0.5 g saturated fat: < 1 g monounsaturated fat: < 1 g cholesterol: 1 mg Sodium: 148 mg potassium: 152 mg Carbohydrates: 28 g Sugar: 10 g dietary fiber: 1.2 g magnesium: 15 mg calcium: 30 mg Iron: 1.5 mg vitamin a: 14 IU vitamin c: < 1 mg

Banana Bread Donuts Honeyed Yogurt Glaze

Servings: 10 (1 donut each)

Ingredients

1/3 cup oat flour 1/2 cup whole wheat flour 3/4 teaspoon baking powder 1/4 teaspoon salt 3/4 teaspoon ground cinnamon two medium bananas, mashed one large egg one medium apple, peeled and grated 1/2 t.

Instructions

1. In a cup, mix the dry ingredients and stir in the banana, potato, apple, and vanilla extract. I am using the mixer to combine it all.
2. Lightly coat the doughnut pan with the cooking spray or vegetable oil and apply the batter. Place in the oven for 20 to 25 minutes or until the toothpick is clean.
3. Remove the doughnuts and let them cool down on the wire rack. Mix yogurt and honey in a small bowl while cooling.
4. When completely cooled, dip the top of each doughnut in the yogurt mixture, making sure to coat the top of each doughnut. Sprinkle on top of the sliced walnuts.
5. You can enjoy it right away or refrigerate for 15 to 20 minutes to allow the glaze to firm up.

Ingredient Combinations and Substitutions

If needed, use full-fat yogurt instead of non-fat yogurt. You're only going to add a few extra calories per doughnut.

You can also give an antioxidant boost to your honeyed yogurt. Heat about 1/4 cup of blueberries before the juices are released, about 3 to 5 minutes on the stovetop with about 1 inch of water or 45 seconds in the microwave, without adding any gas. Let it cool, then whisk in the yogurt mixture before you dip your doughnuts. You should do it with strawberries, too.

Cooking and Serving Tips

If you don't have oatmeal flour, make your own. Place around 1/3 cup oats in the food processor and pulse until finely ground. Make sure you weigh the final product— you may need to add a little more to hit 1/3 cup of the final product.

For a better show, consider grinding your walnuts instead of chopping them. Sprinkle all over the top of the doughnut after you dip it in the yogurt.

You can be flexible with your apple option as long as you pick a sweet one. In the end, the grated and blended apple will turn into apple sauce, so you don't have to worry about the flesh breaking down when you're baking. Excellent options include delicious red, white, fresh honey, and gala apples.

Drink hot tea, cocoa, or matcha latte.

Nutrition Highlights (Per Serving)

100 calories 3 g fat 16 g carbs 4 g protein

6.5 Salads

Our recipes are especially delicious on salads to liven up the taste of

Greens and vegetables

Cranberry Salad

Yield: 8 servings

Ingredients

1 box (3 oz) raspberry Jell-O 1 can make whole cranberry sauce (not jellied) 1 cup apple, peeled and chopped 1 cup celery, chopped 1/2 cup unsalted nuts

Recipe:

1. Mix Jell-O, as instructed by the box.

2. Add cranberry sauce, apple, celery, and nuts when cold and with the consistency of syrup.

3. Chill until strong. Serving cold.

Serve size: 1/2 cup

Per Serving Provides:

Calories: 114 Total fat: 4 g saturated fat: < 1 g monounsaturated fat: 1.1 g polyunsaturated fat: 2.8 g Cholesterol: 0 mg Sodium: 28 mg potassium: 101 mg carbohydrate: 17 g Sugar: 13.5 g total fiber: 1.3 g magnesium: 18 mg calcium: 11 mg vitamin a: 28 IU vitamin c: 1.1 mg vitamin d: 0 µg protein: 2.5 g iron: < 1 mg

Mediterranean Pasta Salad

Yield: 6 servings

Ingredients

4 cups of cooked small macaroni shell 1 tbsp olive oil 2 cups of fresh green beans, 1/2 cup lemon juice 1/3 cup olive oil 2 tsp dry mustard* 1 tbsp fresh parsley, 1 tbsp basil* 1 can of (73/4 oz) salted tuna, drained five green onions, chopped 1/4 tsp pepper*

Recipe:

1. Place pasta in a bowl with 1 tbsp of olive oil and set aside.

2. Blanch the green beans for 2 minutes by dropping them in boiling water.

Switch to a colander and refrigerate under cold water. Drain and drain.

3. Combine beans, lemon juice, 1/3 cup of olive oil, mustard, parsley, and basil into a large pot.

4. Remove fish, green onions, pepper, and pasta. Toss, cover, and then chill for at least 1 or 2 hours before serving.

Serving size: 11/2 cups

Per Serving Provides

Calories: 326 Total fat: 14.5 g saturated fat: 1 g monounsaturated fat: 4.5 g polyunsaturated fat: 9 g Cholesterol: 19 mg Sodium: 64 mg potassium: 265 mg Carbohydrates: 34 g carbohydrates: 34 g Sugar: 1.8 g total fiber: 3.5 g Iron: 2 mg magnesium: 38 mg calcium: 42 mg Protein: 15 protein: 2.5 g vitamin a: 470 IU vitamin c: 18 mg vitamin d: 0 µg iron: < 1 mg

Roasted Vegetable Salad

Yield: 6 servings

Ingredients

12 new potatoes, halved 1 tsp of fresh rosemary, chopped two large red onions, 2 tsp of fresh thyme, chopped* each cut into eight wedges 2 tsp of olive oil two large yellow bell peppers, 1 pint of cherry tomatoes, halved seeds and 1/3 cup toasted pine nuts four cloves of garlic, peeled* 1 sachet of baby spinach leaves one eggplant, thickly sliced 2 tbsp balsamic vinegar

Recipe:

1. Preheat oven to around 400 ° f. Place aluminum foil on a baking sheet.

2. Place the potatoes in a healthy microwave bowl, and put them in the microwave. Cook on high temperature for 3 to 4 minutes until the vegetables are tender.

3. Put the potatoes and the onion, bell pepper, garlic, and eggplant in a large cup. Sprinkle with the olive oil, thyme, and rosemary.

Toss the vegetables with olive oil to coat. You should apply a sodium-free seasoning (such as Mrs. Dash) to taste. Place plants onto a baking sheet prepared.

4. Roast the vegetables in the already heated oven for about 35 minutes, until they start to brown at the edges. Stir in the cherry tomato pieces, and cook for another 15 minutes.

5. Toss the roasted vegetables with the pine nuts, spinach, and balsamic vinegar into a large pot.

Each Serving Provides:

Calories: 215 Total fat: 9.5 g saturated fat: 1 g monounsaturated fat 3.5 g polyunsaturated fat: 5 g Cholesterol: 0 mg Sodium: 67 mg potassium: 982 mg Carbohydrates: 26 g Sugar: 6.8 g total fiber: 8 g Protein: 6.5 g Iron: 5 mg magnesium: 112 mg calcium: 74 mg vitamin a: 2,912 IU vitamin c: 141 mg vitamin d: 0 µg nutrition

Cucumber Couscous Salad

Yield: 8 servings

Ingredients

10 ounces uncooked couscous 2 tbsp olive oil 1/2 cup lemon juice 1/4 tsp salt 1/2 tsp ground black pepper* 1 cucumber, seeded and chopped 1/2 cup of finely chopped green onions 1/2 cup fresh parsley, add chopped 1/4 cup of fresh basil, chopped* 8 leaves lettuce eight slices lemon

Recipe:

1. Take some 13/4 cups of water to a boil in a medium saucepan. Stir the couscous in; cover it. Remove from heat; let stand for 5 minutes, covered.

It was cooling down to room temperature.

2. Meanwhile, mix butter, lemon juice, salt, and pepper in a medium dish. Add cucumber, green onion, parsley, basil, and couscous to taste. Mix well for at least 1 hour, then relax.

3. Fill one plate with leaves of lettuce. Couscous spoon mixture over berries and garnish with wedges of lemon.

Each Serving Provides:

Calories: 186 Total fat: 4 g monounsaturated fat: 2.5 g polyunsaturated fat: 0.5 g saturated fat: 1 g Cholesterol: 0 mg Sodium: 44 mg potassium: 336 mg Carbohydrates: 32 g Sugar: 8 g total fiber: 5.5 g calcium: 78 mg vitamin a: 59 IU vitamin c: 23 mg vitamin d:0 µg iron: 2 mg nutrition

Balsamic Vinaigrette Pasta Salad

Yield: 8 servings

Ingredients

3 cups of pasta of your choice (8 ounces) 2 cups of yellow summer squash, sliced 1 cup of green peas 1/2 red sweet pepper, sliced one can (6 oz) of black olives, drained and chopped 1 cup of cherry tomatoes, halved 1/2 cup of red onion, chopped 2 tsp of dried basil, crushed* 1 cup of balsamic vinaigrette

Recipe:

1. Cook the pasta and drain it. Rinse with cold water, rinse again.

2. Add all of the ingredients in a large bowl and swirl top cover gently.

3. Chill out for 2 to 24 hours and cover.

Each Serving Provides:

Calories: 155 Total fat: 1 g monounsaturated fat: < 1 g polyunsaturated fat: < 1 g saturated fat: < 1 g cholesterol: 0 mg Sodium: 51 mg potassium: 278 mg Carbohydrates: 32 g Sugar: 4 g total fiber: 3,5 g Protein: 3,5 g magnesium: 35 mg calcium: 54 mg Iron: 2 mg vitamin a: 105 IU vitamin c: 29 mg vitamin d: 0 µg nutrition

Blue Cheese and Pear Salad

Yield: 8 servings

Ingredients

1/4 cup sugar 1/2 cup pecans 1/3 cup olive oil 3 1/2 tsp red wine vinegar 1 1/2 tsp mustard 1 clove garlic, 1/4 teaspoon light salt fresh ground black pepper to taste 1 head leaf lettuce, broken in pieces 3 pears, peeled, cored, and diced 3 ounces blue cheese, topped 1/2 cup thinly sliced green onions

Recipe:

1. Stir 1/4 cup of sugar in a skillet over medium heat along with the pecans. Continue stirring it gently until the sugar has melted completely, and the pecans are caramelized. Move the nuts carefully onto waxed paper.

Let it cool down and break into bits.

2. Mix butter, vinegar, 1 1/2 teaspoons of sugar, mustard, chopped garlic, salt, and pepper together for the dressing.

3. Pour lettuce, pears, blue cheese, avocado, and green onions in a large serving dish. Pour over the salad dressing, sprinkle with the pecans, and serve.

Each serving provides:

Calories: 230 Total fat: 15.5 g monounsaturated fat: 10 g polyunsaturated fat: 2 g saturated fat: 3.5 g Cholesterol: 8 mg Sodium: 208 mg potassium: 258 mg carbohydrate: 19 g carbohydrate: 19 g Sugar: 4 g total fiber: 2 g Iron: 0.5 mg magnesium: 19 mg calcium: 77 mg Protein: 3.5 g vitamin a: 48.5 IU vitamin c: 5.5 mg vitamin d: 0 µg nutrition

Caribbean Sweet Potato Salad

Yield: 6 servings

Ingredients

2 large sweet potatoes, peeled and quartered 1 cup corn 1 tsp. Dijon-style mustard 2 tsp. Fresh lime juice 3 tbsp. Fresh cilantro, chopped 1 clove of garlic, minced 3 tbsp. Canola oil 1/4 tsp. Salt 1/4 tsp. Ground black pepper 1 cucumber, halved in length and diced 1/2 red onion, thinly sliced 1/4 cup of finely chopped peanuts

Recipe:

1. Place the pieces of potato in a large casserole, then cover with water.

Bring to a boiler, turn down the heat and simmer for 10-15 minutes. Take a slice of potato, cut it in half to see if it is enough to eat. Once the vegetables are tender, add the kernels of corn; cook for another 30 seconds. Drain over a colander. Fill the casserole with cold water, then put vegetables in broth. Hot, and drain for 5 minutes.

2. Whisk the mustard, lime juice, cilantro, and garlic together in a large cup. Whisk in gasoline, gradually. Mix in black pepper and salt.

3. Break the cooled potatoes into 1-inch cubes, and add the cucumber and red onion to the dressing. Better fire. Serve at or chilled to room temperature. Shortly before eating, put the peanuts in.

Every Serving Provides:

Calories: 184 Total fat: 10 g monounsaturated fat: 5,5 g polyunsaturated fat: 3,5 g saturated fat: 1 g Cholesterol: 0 mg Sodium: 53 mg potassium: 242 mg Carbohydrates: 20 g Sugar: 3 g total fiber: 3,5 g Iron: 0,5 mg vitamin c: 12 mg vitamin d: 0 µg vitamin a: 866 iu magnesium: 35 mg calcium: 22 mg nutrition

Summer Corn and Tomato Salad

Yield: 4 servings

Ingredients

1/4 cup of fresh basil, 3 tbsp of olive oil 2 tsp of lime juice 1 tsp of sugar 1/4 tsp of salt 1/4 tsp of pepper* 2 cups of frozen corn, 2 cups of frozen tomatoes, half a cup of sliced, seeded, peeled cucumber

Recipe:

1. Combine the basil, milk, lime juice, sugar, salt, and pepper in a jar with a tight-fitting lid; stir well.

2. Combine the corn, tomatoes, and cucumber into a full pot.

Drizzle with dressing, then toss to cover. Chill until served.

Each Serving Provides:

Calories: 209 Total fat: 10.5 g monounsaturated fat: 7.5 g polyunsaturated fat: 1.5 g saturated fat: 1.5 g Cholesterol: 0 mg Sodium: 87 mg potassium: 586 mg total fiber: 5 g magnesium: 46 mg calcium: 105 mg vitamin a: 116 IU vitamin c: 25 mg vitamin d: 0 µg iron: 2.5 mg Protein: 3.5 g Sugar: 7 g carbohydrates: 25 g nutrition

Pecan and Avocado Salad

Yield: 1 serving

Ingredients

1 cup baby spinach leaves one tablespoon dried cranberries one tablespoon chopped pecans 1/2 apple, cored and diced one tablespoon diced red onion two tablespoons grated carrot 1/4 avocado, peeled and diced one tablespoon balsamic vinaigrette dressing or to taste

Recipe:

1. Place spinach, cranberries, pecans, apple, onion, carrot, and avocado in a cup. Drizzle with balsamic dressing and flip to cover.

Every Serving Provides

Calories: 253 Total fat: 11.5 g saturated fat: 1.6 g monounsaturated fat: 7.7 g polyunsaturated fat: 2.2 g Cholesterol: 0 mg Sodium: 58 mg potassium: 808 mg carbohydrate: 34 g Sugar: 10 g dietary fiber: 8 g Iron: 2.5 mg magnesium: 79 mg calcium: 78 mg Protein: 3.5 g vitamin a: 795 IU vitamin c: 27 mg vitamin d: 0 µg nutrition

Glazed Parsnip Salad with Pecans

Yield: 6 servings

Ingredients

21/2 cups of a parsnip, cut into thin strips 21/2 cups of carrot, cut into small pieces 1/2 cup of broccoli stems, cut into small pieces 3/4 cup of orange juice 1/2 cup of dried cranberries 1/2 tsp of ground ginger two pears, firm, peeled and sliced 1/3 cup of pecan halves 3 tbsp of brown sugar 2 tbsp of margarine

Recipe:

1. Combine the first six ingredients into a broad skillet. Bring to a boil then rising to medium heat. Cook, uncovered, stirring periodically, for ~6 to 8 minutes. (The bulk of the liquid will evaporate)

2. Add pears, pecans, brown sugar, and margarine to taste. Cook for another 2-3 minutes, uncovered, or until the vegetables are glazed.

Every Serving Provides:

Calories: 325 Total fat: 5.5 g saturated fat: 0.75 g monounsaturated fat: 3 g polyunsaturated fat: 1.8 g Cholesterol: 0 mg Sodium: 54 mg potassium: 611 mg carbohydrate: 42 g Sugar: 12 g dietary fiber: 6.5 Giron: 1.2 mg magnesium: 46 mg calcium: 62 mg Protein: 2.7 g vitamin a: 1.346 IU vitamin c: 49 mg vitamin d:0 µg nutrition

Spinach, Avocado & Mango Salad

Ingredients

Dressing 1/3 cup orange juice one tablespoon red-wine vinegar two tablespoons hazelnut oil, almond oil or canola oil one teaspoon dijon mustard 1/4 teaspoon salt, or to taste salad freshly ground pepper, to taste 1 1/2 cups radicchio, broken in pieces 10 cups baby spinach leaves, (about 8 ounces) 8-12 small red radishes, (1 bunch) sliced one thin slice of radicchio.

Prepare Salad:
1. Mix spinach, radicchio, radishes, and mango in a full bowl just before serving. Attach the cover, throw it to wear. Garnish each serving with slices of avocado.

Nutrition Facts

Serving size: 2 cups per serving: 221 calories; 14.8 g of total fat; 1.7 g of saturated fat; 244 mg sodium. 846 mg of potassium; 22.9 g of carbohydrates; 6.4 g of fiber; 14 g of sugar; 3.7 g of protein; 6345 iu of vitamin iu; 68 mg of vitamin c; 202 mcg of folate; 83 mg of calcium; 2 mg of iron; 72 mg of magnesium; stockings: 3 vegetable, 3 fat (mono)

Crunchy Broccoli Salad

Ingredients

8 cups fresh broccoli flowers (about 1 pound) 1 bunch of green onions, thinly sliced 1/2 cup dried cranberries three tablespoons canola oil three tablespoons seasoned rice vinegar two tablespoons sugar 1/4 cup sunflower kernels three bacon strips, cooked and crumbled

Instructions

1. In a large bowl, mix broccoli, green onions, and cranberries. In a small cup, whisk butter, vinegar, and sugar until blended; drizzle over the broccoli mixture and apply to the coat. Refrigerate until ready to eat. Until serving, sprinkle with sunflower kernels and bacon.

Editor's Note

Wear disposable gloves when cutting hot peppers; oils can burn the skin. Don't touch your nose.

Nutrition Facts

Serves 3/4 cup: 121 calories, 7 g fat (1 g saturated fat), 2 mg cholesterol, 233 mg sodium, 14 g carbohydrate (10 g sugar, 3 g fiber), 3 g protein. Diabetic exchange: 1 grain, one fat, 1/2 starch.

6.6 Soups

Minestrone
Yield: 12 servings
Ingredients
1/4 cup of olive oil 43/4 cups of cabbage, one clove of garlic, 1 pound of minced tomatoes, sliced (or 1/8 tsp of powder)* 1 cup of canned red kidney beans, 11/3 cups of onion, coarsely chopped washed, rinsed 11/2 cups of celery with leaves, 11/2 cups of frozen green peas coarsely chopped 11/2 cups of fresh green beans one can (6 oz) of tomato paste dash hot sauce (not added)

Recipe:
1. Heat the oil in a saucepan for four thirds. Add garlic, onion, and celery, then sauté for 5 minutes.
2. Connect all other ingredients except spaghetti. Cut until the ingredients have mixed properly.
3. Cover and simmer for almost 45 minutes or until the vegetables are tender.
4. Stir in uncooked spaghetti and cook for 2 to 3 minutes.

Every Serving Provides:
Calories: 115 Total fat: 0.5 g saturated fat: 0 g monounsaturated fat: 0.5 g polyunsaturated fat: 0 g Cholesterol: 0 mg Sodium: 189 mg potassium: 467 mg Carbohydrates: 23 g Sugar: 7 g dietary fiber: 5 g magnesium: 32 mg calcium: 62 mg Iron: 2 mg vitamin a: 1.259 IU vitamin c: 26 mg vitamin d: 0 µg nutrition

Turkey Soup with Barley

Yield: 8 to 10 servings

Ingredients

6 pounds turkey breast with bones 1/2 tsp dried sage* (with at least 2 cups of meat) 1 tsp dried basil* 2 medium onions 1/2 tsp dried marjoram three stalks celery 1/2 tsp dried tarragon 1 tsp dried thyme* black pepper at taste* 1/2 tsp dried rosemary 11/2 cups barley

Recipe:
1. Place the turkey breast in a large six-quarter dish. Cover with water to a total of three-quarters maximum.

2. Peel the onions cut them into large pieces, then add them to the bowl. Wash the stalks of celery, sliced, and add them to the pan.

3. Simmer sealed for approximately 21/2 hours.

4. Take carcass out of the pot. Divide the soup into smaller, shallower containers in the refrigerator for fast cooling.

5. Skim off fat, after cooling.

6. Remove extra meat from the turkey carcass as the soup cools.

Split into slices.

7. Add turkey meat, herbs, and spices, to the skimmed broth.

8. Bring to boil and pour in barley. Continue to cook for about 20 minutes on a low boil, until the barley is cooked. Serve immediately or refrigerate for later reheating.

Every Serving Provides:

Calories: 236 Total fat: 2.5 g saturated fat: 1.5 g monounsaturated fat: < 1 g polyunsaturated fat: 1 g Cholesterol: 59 mg Sodium: 68 mg potassium: 407 mg carbohydrate: 27 g Sugar: 5 g dietary fiber: 5.5 g Iron: 2.3 mg magnesium: 50 mg calcium: 44 mg Protein: 26 g vitamin a: 3 mg vitamin d:0 µg nutrition

San Francisco Cioppino

Yield: 8 servings

Ingredients

1/4 cup olive oil one onion, chopped four cloves garlic, minced* 1 green bell pepper, chopped one fresh red chili pepper, seeded and chopped* 1/2 cup fresh parsley salt, to taste Pepper to taste* 2 tsp dried basil* 1 tsp dried oregano 1 tsp dried thyme one can (28 oz) low-crushed tomatoes one can (8 oz) low-tomato.

Recipe:

1. Heat the olive oil in a large pot over medium heat and sauté the onion, garlic, bell pepper, and chili pepper until tender.

2. Add parsley, garlic, basil, oregano, thyme, tomatoes, tomato sauce, sugar, paprika, cayenne pepper, and clam juice.

3. Remove well, may heat, and simmer for 1 to 2 hours, adding some wine at a time.

4. Add clams, mussels, crabs, scallops, and cod about 10 minutes before serving.

5. Turn the heat up and mix. Serve your delicious cioppino when the seafood is cooked through (the mussels should have opened, the shrimp turned pink, and the cod is flaky).

Every Serving Provides:

Calories: 260 Total fat: 7.1 g saturated fat: 1.1 g monounsaturated fat: 4 g polyunsaturated fat: 2 g Cholesterol: 92 mg Sodium: 278 mg potassium: 1012 mg Carbohydrates: 16 g Sugar: 4 g total fiber: 3.3 g Iron: 16 mg vitamin c: 61 mg vitamin d: 7.5 μg magnesium: 98 mg vitamin a: 402 iu nutrition

Cuban Black Bean Soup

Yield: 4 servings

Ingredients

1 pound of dried black beans, rinsed and soaked overnight 1 1/2 cups of low-sodium vegetable broth 1 cup of chopped salsa 1 tsp of ground cumin* 4 tbsp of low-fat sour cream 2 tbsp of green onion, thinly sliced

Recipe:

1. Combine the beans, broth, salsa, and cumin in an electric food processor or blender. Blend in until smooth enough.

2. Heat the bean mixture over medium heat in a saucepan until it heats thoroughly.

3. Ladle soup into four single bowls, and top each bowl with one tablespoon of sour cream and 1/2 tablespoon of green onions.

Every Serving Provides:

Calories: 204 Total fat: 2.2 g monounsaturated fat: 0.5 g saturated fat: 1.2 g Cholesterol: 5 mg Sodium: 388 mg potassium: 176 mg Carbohydrates: 33 g Sugar: 1.2 g dietary fiber: 12.9 g calcium: 53 mg vitamin a: 34 IU vitamin c: 5 mg vitamin d: 0 µg protein: 13 g Iron: 2.5 mg magnesium: 80 mg nutrition

Corn Chowder

Yield: 4 servings

Ingredients

1 tbsp of vegetable oil 2 tbsp of celery, finely diced 2 tbsp of onion, finely diced 2 tbsp of green pepper, finely diced one box (10 oz) of frozen whole kernel corn 1 cup 1/2-inch of raw potatoes, peeled and diced 1 cup of water 1/4 tsp of black salt pepper to taste 1/4 tsp of paprika* 2 cups of low-fat (1%) or skim milk 2 tbsp of fresh parsley 2 tbsp of flour

Recipe:

1. Heat oil in a medium cup.

2. Add 2 minutes of celery, onion, and green pepper, and sauté.

3. Add some corn, potatoes, water, salt, pepper, and paprika to taste. Bring to a boiler; reduce heat to medium, and cook, covered, for around 10 minutes or tender until the potatoes.

4. Layer 1/2 cup milk in a tightly fitted cloth pot. Apply flour and shake briskly.

5. Gradually add to the cooked vegetables and add surplus milk.

6. Cook, continuously stirring until the mixture reaches a boil and thickens. Serve garnished with fresh, chopped parsley.

Each Serving Provides:

Calories: 180 Total fat: 3.5 g monounsaturated fat: 0.5 g polyunsaturated fat: 2.5 g saturated fat: 0.5 g Cholesterol: 2.2 mg Sodium: 146 mg potassium: 577 mg carbohydrate: 30 g Sugar: 4 g total fiber: 2.7 g Iron: 0.8 mg magnesium: 38 mg calcium: mg protein: 7 g vitamin a: 111 IU vitamin c: 13 mg vitamin d: 1.2 µg nutrition

New Orleans Chicken Gumbo with Okra

Yield: 8 servings

Ingredients

8 cups of water 1 tsp of garlic powder 1 tsp of hot pepper sauce two carrots, sliced thin 4 ounces of fresh mushroom one box (10 oz) of frozen okra, roasted and sliced 1/4 cup uncooked wild rice one half of skinless, boneless chicken breast, cut into cubes 11/2 cups of uncooked pasta (rotini) salt to taste ground black pepper to taste*

Recipe:

1. Bring the water to a boil. Connect the garlic powder and the sauce to the hot pepper. Place the carrots and the mushrooms in a bowl of water — cook for five minutes.

2. Attach the okra, the wild rice, the chicken cubes. Switch the heat to low and cook for three hours.

3. Attach the spiral pasta and cook for about 10 minutes. Remove salt and chili pepper to taste. Serve sweet, topped with green onions.

Each Service Shall Provide:

Calories: 142 Total fat: 1.5 g monounsaturated fat: 0.5 g polyunsaturated fat: 0.5 g saturated fat: 0.5 g Cholesterol: 9 mg Sodium: 74 mg potassium: 289 mg carbohydrate:24 g total fiber: 2.5 g Protein: 8 g Iron: 1.8 mg magnesium: 55 mg calcium: 103 mg sugar: 3 g vitamin a: 535 IU vitamin c: 7.7 mg vitamin d: 0.3 µg nutrition

Lentil Soup

Yield: 8 servings

Ingredients

1/4 cup olive oil one onion, chopped two carrots, diced two stalks celery, chopped two cloves garlic, minced 1 tsp dried oregano* 1 bay leaf* (to be extracted after cooking) 1 tsp dried basil 2 cups dried lentils 8 cups water one can (14.5 oz) crushed tomatoes (no added salt) 1/2 cup spinach, rinsed and thinly sliced 2 tsp vinegar salt to taste ground black pepper.

Recipe:

1. Heat oil in a large soup pot over medium heat. Remove ointments, onions, and celery; cook and stir until tender. Incorporate the garlic, oregano, bay leaf, and basil; cook 2 minutes.

2. Remove lentils, then add water and tomatoes. Take to simmer. Reduce flame and simmer for a minimum of 1 hour.

3. Stir in spinach when they are ready to eat, and cook until it wilts. Stir in vinegar and, if necessary, season with salt and pepper to taste, and more vinegar.

Every Serving Provides Calories:

247 total fat: 6,5 g saturated fat: 1 g monounsaturated fat: 5 g polyunsaturated fat: 0,5 g Cholesterol: 0 mg Sodium: 97 mg potassium: 330 mg carbohydrate: 29 g total fiber: 5 g Iron: 12 mg calcium: 110 mg vitamin a: 566 IU vitamin d: 0 µg vitamin c: 15,5 mg sugar: 5 g Protein: 18 g nutrition

Crab and Roasted Corn Soup

Yield: 6 servings

Ingredients

1 box (16 oz) of frozen whole-grain corn 2 cups of chopped onion (2 large) 1½ cups of red sweet pepper, coarsely chopped (3 medium) 1 tbsp of canola oil 4 cans (14 oz each) of low-sodium chicken broth ½ tsp of dried thyme, crushed* ⅛ tsp of cayenne pepper* ⅓ cup of all-purpose flour ½ cup of low-fat sour cream 4 ounces of cooked crabmeat, cut into bite pieces (⅔ cup)

Recipe:

1. Preheat oven to 450 degrees f. frozen corn with the thaw. Pat dry with towels made from cotton. Cover baking pan with foil; grease foil lightly. Place the corn in prepared casserole. Bake 10 minutes in the oven; pour in. Bake, stirring once or twice, for another 10 minutes until golden brown. Switch off the oven; set aside.

2. Cook the onion and sweet pepper in hot oil on medium heat for 3 to 4 minutes or to almost tender in a Dutch oven. Attach roasted maize, three bread crumbs, thyme, and cayenne pepper. Bring to a boil, then reduce for 15 minutes to simmer, uncovered.

3. Combine the remaining can of broth and the flour in a large screw-top pan—cover, and well shaken. Cut to the food. Cook and serve until bubbly and slightly thickened. Stir in the sour cream for 1 minute more than stirring; heat through.

4. Ladle soup in bowls to drink and break crabmeat into cups.

Every Serving Provides:

Calories: 200 Total fat: 4,4 g saturated fat: 1,7 g monounsaturated fat: 1,7 g polyunsaturated fat: 1 g Cholesterol: 25 mg Sodium: 370 mg potassium: 410 mg carbohydrate: 30 g Sugar: 5 g total fiber: 4 g vitamin a: 270 IU vitamin c: 77 mg vitamin d: 0 µg magnesium: 34 mg Protein: 10 g Iron: 11 mg calcium: 73 mg nutrition

6.7 Vegetables or Side Dishes

Green Beans with Slivered Almonds, Garlic, And Basil

Yield: 4 servings

Ingredients

1 1/2 pounds of fresh green beans, 1/3 cup of green onions, one garlic clove, 2 tsp of olive oil 1/4 cup of balsamic vinegar 4 tsp of sugar 1 1/2 tsp of fresh basil* 1/8 tsp of salt 1/4 cup of sliced almonds, toasted

Recipe:

1. Place the beans and cover with water in a saucepan. Bring to a boil; cook for 8 to 10 minutes, uncovered, or until tender.

2. Meanwhile, sauté onions and garlic in oil in a non-stick pan until the onions are tender. Remove the vinegar, basil, sugar, and salt.

Bring it to a boiler; cook until the liquid is halved.

3. Drain the beans; add the mixture to the onions. Cook and stir till warm.

4. Sprinkle over almonds.

Every Serving Provides:

Calories: 159 Total fat: 5 g saturated fat: 0.5 g monounsaturated fat: 3.5 g polyunsaturated fat: 1 g Cholesterol: 0 mg Sodium: 46 mg potassium: 635 mg Carbohydrates: 24 g Sugar: 2 g total fiber: 4.5 g vitamin a: 118 IU vitamin c: 20 mg vitamin d: 0 µg iron: 2.8 mg magnesium: 63 mg calcium: 110 mg nutrition

Moroccan Couscous Pilaf

Yield: 6 servings

Ingredients

1 tbsp of olive oil 1 tbsp of unsalted butter one small onion, cut into 1/4 inch 3/4 tsp of ground cumin* pinch of cayenne pepper one package (10 oz) of medium-grain couscous 1/4 tsp of freshly ground pepper* 2 tbsp of freshly ground parsley, coarsely chopped

Recipe:

1. Bring in a medium saucepan 21/4 cups of water to boil.

2. In the time being, heat the olive oil and butter in a large saucepan over medium-low heat. Remove onions and cook for about 8 minutes, until lightly browned. Stir in cumin and cayenne pepper, then sauté for another 1 minute.

3. Connect the couscous, salt, pepper, and hot water. Cover and simmer over low heat, around 10 minutes, until tender and water are absorbed.

Add peters and drink.

Every Serving Provides:

Calories: 217 Total fat: 4,5 g saturated fat: 1,5 g monounsaturated fat: 2,2 g polyunsaturated fat: < 1 g cholesterol: 5 mg Sodium: 55 mg potassium: 184 mg carbohydrate: 38 g Sugar: 10 g total fiber: 2,5 g vitamin a: 26 IU vitamin d: 0 μg vitamin c: 3 mg Protein: 6 g Iron: 0,5 mg magnesium: 24 mg calcium: 18 mg nutrition

Autumn Succotash

Yield: 6 servings

Ingredients

1 pack (10 oz) frozen lima beans 1 pack (10 oz) frozen whole-grain corn 2 small tomatoes, 1/4 cup green onion, 1/4 tsp fresh parsley, 1/4 cup red wine 2 tbsp Italian salad dressing 1/4 tsp dry mustard*

Recipe:

1. Cook lima beans and corn as directed by package; drain. Combine lima beans, peas, tomatoes, green onion, and parsley in a dish.

2. Whisk together the red wine vinegar, sauce, and mustard in a small mixing cup. Pour over a mixture of Lima beans; flip to cover. Serve at or chilled to room temperature.

Serving size: 1/2 cup

Per Serving Provides:

Calories: 119 Total fat: 3 g saturated fat: 0,5 g monounsaturated fat: 1 g polyunsaturated fat: 1,5 g Cholesterol: 0 mg Sodium: 30 mg potassium: 332 mg Carbohydrates: 19 g Sugar: 4 g total fiber: 4 g vitamin c: 14 mg vitamin d:0 µg vitamin a: 38 IU vitamin a: 38 IU vitamin a: 38 iu iron: 1 mg magnesium: 28 mg calcium: 17 mg nutrition

Mediterranean Orzo Pasta

Yield: 6 servings

Ingredients

3 quarts of water 11⁄3 cups (8 oz) of dry orzo pasta 2 tsp of olive oil one clove of garlic, 1⁄2 tsp of Italian seasoning (marjoram bleach, thyme, rosemary, savory, sage, oregano, and basil) 1 tbsp parmesan cheese, grated

Recipe:

1. Bring to boil tea. Attach orzo, and pour in water. Return to a boil and cook for 9 to 11 minutes or until cooked, uncovered (eviting overcooking for better results).

2. Remove from heat and drain in colander well.

3. Pour drained pasta into a bowl to eat. Connect olive oil, garlic, parmesan cheese, and Italian seasoning. Gently throw in and serve.

Every Serving Provides:

Calories: 128 Total fat: 2 g saturated fat: 0.5 g monounsaturated fat: 1.25 g polyunsaturated fat: < 1 g cholesterol: 0.8 g Sodium: 21 mg potassium: 42 mg Carbohydrates: 25 g Sugar: 8 g dietary fiber: 0.5 g Iron: 1.1 mg vitamin d: 0 µg vitamin a: 2.6 IU vitamin c: < 1 mg protein: 2.5 g magnesium: 10.5 mg calcium: 35 mg nutrition

Broccoli-Cauliflower-Carrot Bake

Yield: 12 servings

Ingredients

3 cups of broccoli, raw 2 cups of cauliflower, fresh 1 cup of frozen whole small onions or three medium onions, quartered 1 cup of carrots, chopped 4 tbsp of butter 2 tbsp of flour 1/4 tsp of black pepper* 1 cup of fat-free milk one box (3 oz) of cream cheese, softened 1/2 cup of cheddar cheese, shredded 1/2 cup of soft breadcrumbs

Recipe:

1. Wash and cut the vegetables; steam until soft yet crisp. Drain and drain.

2. Melt 2 tbsp of butter in the saucepan; stir in flour and pepper.

Add milk, and cook/stir until thick and bubbly.

3. Reduce heat and mix until smooth in cream cheese.

4. Place the vegetables in an 11/2-quarter casserole dish, then pour over the sauce and mix well. Cover with whipped cheese.

5. Bake at 350 ° f for 15 minutes.

6. In the meantime, mix the breadcrumbs and remaining butter, then sprinkle on the casserole and bake for another 25 minutes.

Each Serving Provides:

Calories: 132 Total fat: 7.5 g monounsaturated fat: 2.3 g polyunsaturated fat: <1 g saturated fat: 4.5 g Cholesterol: 21 mg Sodium: 163 mg potassium: 260 mg Carbohydrates: 11 g carbohydrates: <1 g total fiber: 2 g Iron: 1 mg vitamin c: 31 mg vitamin d: 0.5 µg vitamin a: 455 iu protein: 5 g magnesium: 19 mg calcium: 193 mg nutrition

Roasted Sweet Potatoes

Yield: 6 servings

Ingredients

2 large sweet potatoes, peeled and cut into1-inch 2 medium Vidalia or other sweet onions, chopped into1-inch 3 tbsp olive oil 1/4 cup amaretto liqueur 1 tsp dried thyme freshly ground black pepper to taste* 1/4 cup sliced almonds, toasted

Recipe:

1. Heat oven to 425 ° f.

2. Throw the first six ingredients into a medium-sized, shallow baking dish.

3. Cover; simmer for 30 minutes. Uncover; bake for another 20 minutes.

4. Sprinkle with almonds

Each Serving Provides:

Calories: 159 Total fat: 8.5 g monounsaturated fat: 6.1 g polyunsaturated fat: 1.2 g saturated fat: 1.2 g Cholesterol: 0 mg Sodium: 10 mg potassium: 211 mg carbohydrate: 18 g Sugar: 6 g total fiber: 2.5 g Iron: 0.5 mg vitamin c: 13 mg vitamin d: 0 µg vitamin a: 858 iu magnesium: 22.5 mg calcium: 32.5 mg

Roasted Acorn Squash

Yield: 2 servings

Ingredients

1 medium acorn squash, halved and seeded 1 tbsp butter 2 tbsp brown sugar

Recipe:

1. Preheat oven to 350 degrees f.

2. Turn upside down acorn squash onto a cookie sheet — bake in a 350 ° f oven for about 30 to 45 minutes before it starts to soften.

3. Remove squash from the oven and turn it onto a plate for the flesh to face upwards. Place butter and brown sugar in the squash, and on the other piece, put the remaining squash. Put squash in a baking dish (so the squash isn't going to slip too much around), when baking.

4. Place squash in the oven at 350 ° f and bake for another 30 minutes.

Each Serving Provides:

Calories: 262 Total fat: 6 g monounsaturated fat: 1,7 g polyunsaturated fat: <1 g saturated fat: 3,5 g Cholesterol: 15 mg Sodium: 73 mg potassium: 1,120 mg carbohydrate: 49 g Sugar: 12 g total fiber: 10,5 g Iron: 2,5 mg vitamin a: 159 IU vitamin d: 0 µg vitamin c: 26 mg calcium: 121 mg Protein: 3 g magnesium: 109 mg nutrition

Crispy Edamame

Yield: 8 servings

Ingredients

1 box (12 oz) of frozen edamame (green soybeans) 1 tbsp of olive oil 1/4 cup of parmesan cheese, pepper grated to taste*

Recipe:

1. Preheat oven to 400 degrees f.

2. Thaw edamame in a colander under the cold spray. Drain and drain.

3. Place edamame beans into a 9-by-13-inch baking dish and drizzle with olive oil to the rim. Sprinkle the cheese over the top and pepper to season.

4. Bake until the cheese is crisp (~15 minutes) and golden.

Every Serving Provides:

Calories: 106 Total fat: 6 g saturated fat: 1.3 g monounsaturated fat: 2.4 g polyunsaturated fat: 2.3 g Cholesterol: 2.5 g Sodium: 59 mg potassium: 223 mg Carbohydrates: 5 g sugar: < 1 g dietary fiber: 2.5 g magnesium: 38 mg vitamin d: 0 µg vitamin a: 5.8 iu calcium: 86 mg Protein: 8 g Iron: 2.2 mg vitamin c: 0.7 mg nutrition

Spinach Spaghetti Aglio E Olio

Servings: 2 (1 cup each)

Nutrition Facts (Per Serving)

290 calories 8 g fat 45 g carbs 10 g protein

Ingredients

4 oz dry spaghetti four garlic cloves, sliced 1/2 cup parsley leaves, minced one tablespoon olive oil 1/2 cup spinach leaves, diced 4 oz.

Note

Don't forget to salt the water and focus on preparing the other ingredients while the spaghetti is on the burner.

Instructions

1. Heat the olive oil in a medium saucepan over low heat. Connect the garlic and red pepper flakes and sauté for about 2 minutes.
2. Attach the cooked and drained spaghetti to the skillet and mix until combined with oil and garlic.

3. Attach the parsley and spinach, whisk until well blended. Let it cook for 2 minutes more before turning off the heat and plating.

Ingredient Variations and Substitutions

You can use a particular form of pasta— fettuccine, linguine, macaroni or penne— in equivalent quantities (4 ounces). Certain dark leafy greens, such as kale, collards, or swiss chards, would also fit.

Cooking and Serving Tips

This is the ideal side dish for freshly roasted chicken or salmon (if you have time). Leftovers are working, too.

You can eat the dish on your own, too. Even if you're an essential meal, you can improve the presentation to make it more enjoyable. Using a beautiful plate, garnish with some extra parsley leaves, and try to eat while you enjoy every bite.

Lemon Couscous with Broccoli

Ingredients

1 tablespoon of olive oil 4 cups of fresh broccoli flowers, cut into small pieces 1 cup of uncooked whole-wheat couscous two garlic cloves, minced

Instructions

1. Remove the broccoli; cook and stir until crisp.
2. Add couscous and garlic; cook and stir for 1-2 minutes. Stir in the water, lemon zest, lemon juice, and seasoning; bring to a boil. Remove from heat; let stand, cover until the broth is absorbed for 5-10 minutes. It's fluff with a pin. Sprinkle with some almonds.
3. Toast nuts, bake in a 350 ° oven in a shallow pan for 5-10 minutes or cook in a skillet over low heat until lightly browned, stirring occasionally.

Nutrition Facts

Serves 2/3 cup: 115 calories, 3 g fat (0 saturated fat), 0 cholesterol, 328 mg sodium, 18 g carbohydrate (1 g sugar, 4 g fiber), 5 g protein. Diabetic exchange: 1 starch, 1/2 fat.

Spinach' n' Broccoli Enchiladas

Ingredients

1 medium onion, two teaspoons olive oil one box (10 ounces) frozen chopped spinach, 1 cup finely chopped fresh broccoli 1 cup Picante sauce, 1/2 teaspoon garlic powder 1/2 teaspoon ground cumin 1 cup daisy 1 percent cottage cheese 1 cup diced cheddar cheese, eight flour tortillas 8 oz.

Instructions

1. In a large nonstick pot over the medium heat, cook and stir in the oil until tender. Add spinach, broccoli, 1/3 cup of Picante sauce, garlic powder, and cumin; heat through.
2. Remove from heat; stir in cheddar cheese and 1/2 cup cheddar cheese. Spoon about 1/3 cup of spinach mixture down the middle of each tortilla. Roll up and put the seam side in a 13x9-in. Cooking dish sprayed with a cooking mist. Spoon the remaining piquant sauce over the rim.
3. Cover and bake for 20-25 minutes or until the mixture are heated. Uncover it; sprinkle with the remaining cheese. Bake for 5 minutes or until cheese is melted.

Nutrition Details

1 enchilada: 246 calories, 8 g fat (3 g saturated fat), 11 mg cholesterol, 614 mg sodium, 32 g carbohydrate (4 g sugar, 2 g fiber), 13 g protein. Diabetic exchange: 1-1/2 starch, one lean meat, one potato, 1/2 fat.

Gluten-Free Treat: Flourless Peanut Butter Chocolate Chip Cookies

servings: 24 (1 cookie each)

Ingredients

1 cup of natural peanut butter 3/4 cup of light brown sugar one large egg, one teaspoon of baking soda one teaspoon of vanilla extract 1/2 cup of the mint chocolate chip with coarse sea salt

Preparation

1. Preheat oven to 350f.
2. Cover a sheet of parchment paper or silicone baking pad.
3. In a medium bowl, mix peanut butter and sugar until well blended.
4. Add sugar, baking soda, and vanilla extract; continue stirring until all ingredients are well blended.
5. Layer the chocolate chips.
6. Using a small ice cream scoop or a teaspoon, measure eight cookies in the prepared sheet pan, leaving about two inches between each cookie.
7. Push gently to flatten each cookie slightly.
8. Bake for 6 to 8 minutes until it is puffed and spread out.
9. Remove from the oven and sprinkle lightly with sea salt.
10. Using a spatula, switch to a wire rack to cool down.
11. When completely cooled, store in an airtight jar for up to 2 days.

Ingredient Combinations and Substitutions

You can inject various flavors into these cookies by replacing the vanilla extract with 1/4 teaspoon of extra almond or by changing the chocolate chips for finely chopped peanuts.

Cooking and Serving Tips

Mix the dough by hand with a sturdy spatula or using an electric stand mixer with a paddle attachment. Cookies spread out quite a bit, so it's better to make three batches of 8 if you're using a regular half-leaf pan. Using a small ice cream scoop is very helpful to make cookies equally shaped so that they cook evenly.

Nutrition Highlights (Per Serving)

111 calories 7 g fat 11 g carbs 3 g protein beef in red wine ingredients 800 g beef diced, casserole or rind 3-carrots, sliced 8-mushrooms, quartered two onions sliced five cloves of garlic, crushed 2 cups of red wine, shiraz or cab sav 2 cups of beef stock (water powdered) 2 tbsp. Olive oil one tomato can be diced one small tomato paste 1 tbsp. Brown sugar dried thyme and oregano salt and pepper 2 tbsp. Corn flour mixed with 1/2 cup cold water six large potatoes, boiled and ground with milk, s & p procedure we used a slow cooker, or you can use the oven, 150c.

Heat the olive oil in a frypan and sauté the onions for 10 minutes over low heat. Place in a slow cooker or casserole dish when cooking.

Fry the same pan, brown the meat in 2 batches and put it on top of the onions.

Add wine, garlic, sugar stock, spices, canned tomatoes, purée of vegetables, and season with s&p. Set it down for 4 hours.

After 4 hours, add carrots and mushrooms, add cornflour and a mixture of water and cook for another 4 hours.

Serve with the mashed potatoes.

Serving size: 528 g energy 1800 KJ protein 38.4 g total fat 15.6 g saturated fat 5 g carbohydrate 25 g sugar 9.8 g sodium 173

Cauliflower Mash

Calories 41 per serving protein 4 g per serving

Per serving serves 6

Ingredients

1 medium head cauliflower, cut into flowers (about 6-cups) 3 tablespoon parmesan cheese 1/4 cup plain, fat-Greek yogurt 1/2 teaspoon minced garlic pepper (to a cup)

Instructions

1. In a full pot of about 2 inches of water, cook the cauliflower in a steamer pan, if possible, for about 15 minutes or until tender. Okay, drain, okay.
2. In a blender, food processor or blender, purée the cauliflower with yogurt, parmesan cheese, and garlic until creamy (don't over-mix). To taste the pepper.
3. Serve with pork chops pizza

Fast tip: serve with pork chops pizza recipe!

Calories 41 per serving, protein 4 g per serving

Roasted Parmesan and Almond Cauliflower

Time 10 minutes

Cooking time 30 minutes

Serve 4

Ingredients

1 broad flower head (about 750 g/1 1/2 lb), cut into flowers 125 g (1/2 c) raisins 75 g (1/3 c) pure dried bread crumbs 30 ml (2 tbsp) grated parmesan cheese 15 ml (1 tbsp) sliced almonds 10 ml (2 tsp) olive oil 30 ml (2 tbsp) fresh lemon juice

Instructions

1. Preheat the oven at 200 ° c or 400 °f. Cover large toast pan with foil and spray foil with nonstick cooking spray. Cook the cauliflower in a steamer over a boiling water pan until crisp, about 5 minutes. Move the flower to the roasting pan.

2. In the meantime, add the raisins, the bread crumbs, the parmesan, the almonds, and the butter in a medium dish.

3. Sprinkle the bread crumbs over the cauliflower. Roast the cauliflower until the crumbs are toasted for about 20 minutes. Drizzle the lemon juice on top and roast for 5 minutes. Serve hot or moist at room temperature.

Primary Nutrients:

170 calories, 40 calories from fat, 5 g fat, 1 g saturated fat,0 g trans fat, 6 g protein, 32 g sugar, 5 g fiber, 130 mg sodium blood pressure nutrients: 117 mg vitamin c, 41 mg magnesium, 581 mg potassium, 91 mg calcium

6.8 Entrees

Polynesian Turkey Kabobs

Yield: 15 servings

Ingredients

1 pound lean ground turkey, 1/3 cup unsalted crackers, 1/4 cup liquid egg substitute 1/4 cup ointment, 1 tsp ground ginger* 1 garlic clove, one can (20 oz) pineapple chunks in water, one large red bell pepper one large green bell pepper 1/3 cup reserved pineapple water 2 tbsp margarine, melted 2 tbsp orange marmalade 1½ tsp ground ginger*

Recipes:

1. Place the first six ingredients into a medium dish. Shape into meatballs.

2. Arrange meatballs with pineapple chunks and pepper bits on fifteen8-inch skewers, and put them on the broiler plate.

3. Stir the pineapple juice, margarine, marmalade, and ginger in a small bowl until blended. Brush kabobs over.

4. Broil for 20 minutes 4 inches from the heat source, turn once and baste with sauce.

Each Serving Provides:

Calories: 90 Total fat: 2 g monounsaturated fat: 0.5 g polyunsaturated fat: 0.7 g saturated fat: 0.8 g Cholesterol: 21.5 g Sodium: 73 mg potassium: 110 mg Carbohydrates: 9.9 g Sugar: 7 g total fiber: 1 g calcium: 23 mg vitamin c: 35.8 mg vitamin d: 0 µg vitamin a: 599.05 iu magnesium: 5.37 mg Iron: 0.87 mg Protein: 8 g nutrition

Spinach Lasagna

Yield: 10 servings

Ingredients

1 yellow onion, chopped two cans (14.5 oz each) of whole tomatoes (no salt added), cut two boxes (6 oz each) of tomato paste (low sodium) 2 cups of water 1 tsp of parsley, chopped 1 tsp of salt 1 tsp of garlic powder and 1/2 tsp of black pepper* 1 tsp of basil* 1 bay leaf (to be extracted after cooking sauce) 1/2 tsp of oregano* 1 box of frozen chopped spinach (defrost in microwaves).

Recipe:

1. Sauté the onion in a big, heavy oven. The light brown and drain. Add tomatoes, rice, sugar, parsley, salt, powdered garlic, pepper, basil, bay leaf, and oregano. Simmer, stirring regularly, uncovered, about 30 minutes, then apply drained spinach.

2. While the noodles are cooked as directed; drain. Alternate layers of noodles, sauces, cottage cheese, mozzarella, spinach lasagna, and parmesan cheese — repeat in big, long casserole dish; you'll have three layers. Do not place the cottage cheese on the top sheet it's going to burn).

3. Bake for 40 to 50 minutes at 350 ° f until lightly browned and bubbling. Let stand for 15 minutes; cut to serving in squares.

Each Serving Provides:

Calories: 343 Total fat: 7 g monounsaturated fat: 2 g polyunsaturated fat: 0,5 g saturated fat: 4,5 g Cholesterol: 20 mg Sodium: 600 mg potassium: 940 mg carbohydrate: 47 g carbohydrate: 7 g total fiber: 6 g calcium: 401 mg vitamin a: 2,567 IU vitamin c: 32 mg vitamin d: 0 µg magnesium: 81 mg Iron: 2,5 mg Protein: 23 g nutrition

Omelet Casserole

Yield: 8 servings

Use the egg replacement for a lower cholesterol version and play with extra-nutritional vegetables such as sliced mushrooms, bell peppers, and tomatoes.

Ingredients

4 cups of whole wheat bread, cubed 1 1/2 cups of shredded Swiss cheese (low sodium) 2 cups of egg substitute 3 cups of fat-free (skim) milk 1/2 teaspoon salt 3/4 teaspoon Worcestershire sauce 3/4 cup of onion, 1/8 cup of roasted red bell pepper 1/8 cup of green bell pepper four slices of cooked turkey bacon, 1 cup of chopped fresh basil* sliced pepper to taste*

Recipe:

1. Grease baking dish, 9-by-12-inch. Arrange slices of bread on the bottom of the plate and sprinkle with cheese.

2. Mix the eggs, salt, milk, and Worcestershire sauce. To the egg mixture, add garlic, red and green pepper, turkey bacon, and basil. Garnish over bread and cheese. Season with to taste pepper.

3. Cover it and let it chill for 1 to 2 hours, or overnight.

4. Preheat oven to 325 degrees f. Bake for 50 to 60 minutes until the top is golden, with eggs set. Cut, and serve, into eight squares.

Every Serving Provides:

Calories: 262 Total fat: 10 g saturated fat: 5 g monounsaturated fat: 3 g Cholesterol: 31 mg Sodium: 676 mg potassium: 474 mg carbohydrate: 20 g Sugar: 8 g total fiber: 2.5 g magnesium: 31 mg calcium: 470 mg vitamin a: 877 iu vitamin c: 8 mg vitamin d: 1 µg protein: 23 g nutrition

Salmon Almandine

Yield: 2 servings

Ingredients

2 (4-ounce servings) skinless salmon filets 2 tbsp margarine 3 tbsp sliced almonds 1½ tsp freshly squeezed lemon juice 2 tsp freshly chopped parsley

Recipe:

1. Preheat oven to 400 degrees f.

2. Sprinkle generously on an 8-by-8-inch baking pan with cooking spray. Place salmon fillets in a saucepan and bake for 10 to 15 minutes.

3. Prepare the sauce while baking fish fillets.

4. Melt the margarine over medium heat in a small saucepan. Remove the almonds, then sauté until golden brown (about 8 minutes).

Stir repeatedly.

5. Remove pan from oil, add lemon juice and stir gently.

6. Place the cooked salmon on plates to eat. Pour over the salmon sauce and garnish with the chopped parsley.

Serving size: 1 4-ounce fish fillet

Per Serving Provides

Calories: 233 Total fat: 13 g saturated fat: 3 g monounsaturated fat: 7 g polyunsaturated fat: 3 g Cholesterol: 25 mg Sodium: 548 mg potassium: 349 mg Carbohydrates: 6 g Sugar: 1 g total fiber: 2 g Iron: 1.3 mg calcium: 46 mg Protein: 23 g vitamin a: 468 IU vitamin c: 3.5 mg magnesium: 1.2 mg

Lemon Tarragon Chicken

Yield: 12 servings

Ingredients

2 tbsp margarine eight medium-, boneless chicken breast half (approximately 1½ pounds) 2 fresh mushrooms, halved two garlic cloves, minced 3 tbsp dry sherry ½ tsp dry tarragon, crushed ½ tsp lemon pepper seasoning ¼ cup low-⅓ cup flour ¼ cup light sour cream egg noodles or pasta of your choice.

Recipe:

1. melt margarine over medium heat in a 12-inch skillet. Seasoning with the chicken, onions, garlic, sherry, tarragon, and lemon pepper. Cook for 10-12 minutes, uncovered, or until chicken is no longer pink.

2. Drop slotted spoon with chicken and mushrooms.

3. Combine chicken broth and flour in a screw-top jar and mix well until blended. Attach the skillet and cook mixture, and stir over medium-high heat until the mixture is thick and bubbling.

4. Take from the skillet about half of the mixture, then whisk in sour cream. Return to skillet followed by chicken and mushrooms. Pour in, but don't boil.

5. Serve over cooked noodles that are soft.

Every Serving Provides:

Calories: 223 Total fat: 3 g saturated fat: 1 g monounsaturated fat: 1.5 g polyunsaturated fat: 0.5 g Cholesterol: 64 mg Sodium: 426 mg potassium: 95 mg carbohydrate: 32 g sugar: < 1 g total fiber: 1.5 g Iron: 2.5 mg magnesium: 24 mg calcium: 24 mg Protein: 17 g vitamin a: 115 IU vitamin c: 2.8 mg vitamin d: 0.4 mg nutrition

Spanish Chicken and Shrimp Paella

Yield: 8 servings

Ingredients

1 cup long-1 pound long-chicken breast, cut into 1/2 inch pieces 1/4 cup olive oil one can (10 1/2 oz) low-1/2 pound medium-shrimp, peeled and cleaned 1/2 cup frozen green peas 1/3 cup red bell pepper, chopped 1/3 cup green onion, thinly sliced 1/3 cup yellow onion, chopped two garlic peas, ¼ tsp black pepper, ¼ tsp ground saffron

Recipe:

1. Cook rice, then set it aside.

2. In a two-quarter casserole dish, mix rice, olive oil, and broth with a lid, for 4 to 5 minutes of microwave on high.

3. Attach shrimp, peas, pepper bell, onions, garlic, black pepper, and saffron. Cover and microwave for 3 1/2 to 4 1/2 minutes on high, or until the shrimp turns orange.

4. Stir in the rice which is cooked. Cover and let stand and then serve for 5 minutes.

Serving size: half cup

Each Serving Provides:

Calories: 139 Total fat: 2.5 g monounsaturated fat: 1.5 g polyunsaturated fat: 0.5 g saturated fat: 0.5 g Cholesterol: 70 mg Sodium: 400 mg potassium: 173 mg Carbohydrates: 10 g carbohydrates: 10 g Sugar: 1.5 g total fiber: 1 g Iron: 1.5 mg vitamin c: 22.5 mg vitamin d: 0 µg calcium: 30 mg Protein: 19 g magnesium: 20 mg vitamin a: 621 iu

Spicy Santa Fe Chicken Fajitas

Yield: 10 servings

Ingredients

1 pound of boneless chicken breast 1/4 tsp of pepper* 1 clove of garlic, 1 tsp of chili powder 2 tbsp of lime juice 1 tbsp of fresh cilantro, 1 tbsp of canola oil 1 cup of tomato, 2 tbsp of fresh cilantro, chopped 1 tbsp of red onion, chopped 1/4 tsp of garlic, minced ten flour tortillas (7-inch) 3 cups of lettuce shredded, ½ cup light sour cream

Recipe:

1. Sprinkle with peppered chicken, one hazelnut garlic, chili powder, lime juice, 1 tbsp cilantro, and butter. Switch to model. Cover and marinate for 3 hours or longer in the refrigerator.

2. Combine the tomato, 2 tbsp of cilantro, onion, and 1/4 tsp of garlic in a small bowl to produce salsa. Let them stand for 1 hour.

3. Broil the chicken at each side for 10 minutes, 6 inches from the fire. Split to stripes. Cover tortillas in aluminum foil and fire them up in the oven for 8 minutes as the chicken cooks.

4. Wrap chicken, salsa, lettuce, and sour cream into warm tortillas to eat.

Every Serving Provides:

Calories: 286 Total fat: 6 g saturated fat: 2 g monounsaturated fat: 3 g polyunsaturated fat: 1 g Cholesterol: 25 mg Sodium: 624 mg potassium: 199 mg Carbohydrates: 42 g carbohydrates: < 1 g total fiber: 3 g Iron: 2.9 mg vitamin c: 7 mg vitamin d: 0 µg calcium: 50 mg Protein: 16 g magnesium: 24 mg vitamin a: 120 iu nutrition

Asian Pork-Fried Rice

Yield: 6 servings

Ingredients

3 tbsp canola oil two cloves of garlic, minced 1/4 cup green onion, chopped 2/3 cup carrot, chopped 1/2 cup pork loin, chopped 4 cups of rice 1 tsp low sodium soy sauce 1/2 cup frozen green peas 11/2 cups low cholesterol egg substitute, scrambled and cut 1/4 tsp dry mustard*

Recipe:

1. Heat the oil on medium heat level in a large skillet. Attach the garlic and simmer until smooth. Stir in carrot and onion and cook for 2 minutes.

2. Include pork, pasta, and sauce made with soya. Remove and boil for 3 minutes.

3. Add remaining ingredients and simmer until thoroughly cooked.

Serve size: 1 cup

Each Serving Provides:

Calories: 277 Total fat: 7,2 g saturated fat:0,7 g monounsaturated fat: 4,5 g polyunsaturated fat: 2 g Cholesterol: 8 mg Sodium: 180 mg potassium: 218 mg carbohydrate: 39 g Sugar: 2 g total fiber: 1 g Iron: 3 mg calcium: 32 mg vitamin a: 1,816 IU vitamin c: 4 mg vitamin d: 1 µg magnesium: 21 mg Protein: 14 g nutrition

Louisiana-Shrimp Creole

Yield: 4 servings

Ingredients

1 pound fresh or frozen medium shrimp in shells 3/4 cup chopped onion one stalk chopped celery 3/4 cup green bell pepper, chopped two cloves garlic 2 tbsp canola oil one can (14.5 oz) chopped tomatoes (low sodium), add undrained 1/4 tsp cayenne pepper, add 1/8 tsp salt, 1/2 tsp paprika* 1 tbsp fresh parsley 2 cups cooked rice

Recipe:

1. Shrimp peel and devein, remove ears. Rinse and dry pat; put aside.

2. Cook onion, celery, bell pepper, and garlic over medium heat in a large skillet in hot oil for ~5 minutes or until tender. Add undrained tomatoes, cayenne pepper, salt, and paprika to taste. Bring to boil, then heat down and cook, uncovered, for 5 to 8 minutes or until thickened.

3. Stir in the mixture, shrimp, and parsley. Stir sometimes for 2-4 minutes or until shrimp is finished — season with rice.

Every Serving Provides:

Calories: 259 Total fat: 7 g saturated fat: 0,4 g monounsaturated fat: 4 g polyunsaturated fat: 2,5 g Cholesterol: 134 mg Sodium: 212 mg potassium: 555 mg carbohydrate: 31 g Sugar: 6 g total fiber: 2.5 g Iron: 4 mg vitamin c: 47 mg vitamin d: 2.5 µg protein: 18 g magnesium: 52 mg calcium: 82 mg vitamin a: 214 iu nutrition

Sealed Garlic Scallops

Yield: 4 servings

Ingredients

1 pound of fresh or frozen sea scallops three cloves of garlic, 1 tbsp of butter 2 tbsp of dry white wine 1 tbsp of new chives.

Recipe:

1. If frozen, then thaw scallops. Rinse the scallops and dry hold.

2. In a pan, cook the garlic over medium-high heat in 1/2 tbsp melted butter for 30 seconds. Attach scallops.

3. Cook for 2 to 4 minutes, stirring regularly or until the scallops become opaque. Remove from the skillet and switch to a platter for serving.

4. Fill the skillet with the remaining 1/2 tbsp butter and juice. Cook and mix to let any brown bits loose. Pour the scallops over; sprinkle with the chives.

Every Serving Provides:

Calories: 138 Total fat: 5,5 g saturated fat: 2,5 g monounsaturated fat: 2 g polyunsaturated fat: 1 g Cholesterol: 44 mg Sodium: 539 mg potassium: 339 mg carbohydrate: 3,5 g Sugar: 0 g total fiber: 0 g calcium: 34 mg vitamin c: 4 mg vitamin d:0,1 µg protein: 18,5 g Iron: 0,4 mg magnesium: 62 mg nutrition

Vegetable-Flounder Bake

Yield: 4 servings

Ingredients

1 pound flounder fillets 2 tsp of lemon zest *(~3/4 inch thick) 1/2 tsp of dried oregano* 2 cups of carrots, sliced thin, 1/8 tsp of salt, lightly cooked 1/4 tsp of black pepper* 2 cups of fresh mushroom, sliced 4 cloves of garlic, halved 1/2 tsp of olive oil, 1/2 cup of green onion, chopped 2 small oranges, sliced thin

Recipe:

1. Rinse fish and dry hold. Cut into four pcs.

2. Cut four pieces of thick aluminum foil, 24 inches long. Fold in half each and make four 18-by-12-inch sets.

3. Combine carrots, zucchini, green onion, lemon zest, oregano, salt, pepper, mushrooms, and garlic in a large cup.

4. Divide the vegetables into four pieces of foil, place them in the middle of the foil. Place one piece of flounder fillet over every portion of the plant.

5. Drizzle the 1/2 tsp olive oil over each slice of flounder. Top with orange slices and seal with double folding foil. Ensure sure all edges of the foil are entirely sealed, allowing steam room to create. Place the foiled vegetable-flounder bake on a baking pan.

6. Bake for ~20 to 30 minutes at 350 ° f, or until fish flakes with a fork. Carefully open the foil allowing steam to escape.

Each Serving Provides:

Calories: 239 Total fat: 7 g monounsaturated fat: 4 g polyunsaturated fat: 2 g saturated fat: 1 g Cholesterol: 49 mg Sodium: 305 mg potassium: 217 mg carbohydrate: 18 g total fiber: 4 g Protein: 26 g Iron: 1.1 mg calcium: 80 mg vitamin c: 4.8 mg vitamin d:0 µg sugar: 12 g vitamin a: 0 iu nutrition

Caribbean Roughy

Yield: 4 servings

Ingredients

11/2 pounds orange rough 1/4 cup fresh cilantro 1 tsp lime zest 11/4 tsp lime juice 1 tbsp butter, melted black pepper to taste*

Recipe:

1. Break the fish into four pieces in serving format.

2. Place fish on a grated broiler saucepan. Broil until fish flakes. (Allow fish thickness of 4 to 6 minutes per 1/2-inch.)

3. In the meantime, mix the cilantro, lime zest, lime juice, melted butter in a small cup.

4. Cilantro spoon put together over fish and serve.

Each Serving Provides:

Calories: 156 Total fat: 4 g monounsaturated fat: 2 g polyunsaturated fat: 0 g saturated fat: 2 g Cholesterol: 42 mg Sodium: 258 mg potassium: 175 mg Carbohydrates: 2 g carbohydrates:0 g total fiber: 0 g Iron: 1.2 mg calcium: 50 mg vitamin c: 3 mg vitamin d:0 µg protein: 28 g magnesium: 18 mg vitamin a: 0 iu nutrition

Vegetable Orzo

Yield: 4 servings

Ingredients

1 tbsp of olive oil, 1 cup uncooked orzo pasta one clove garlic, crushed one medium zucchini, shredded one medium carrot, shredded 1can (14 oz) low-sodium vegetable broth one lemon, zested (or zested one lemon), 1 tbsp fresh thyme, chopped 1/4 cup grated parmesan cheese

Recipe:

1. Heat up the oil over medium heat in a kettle. Stir in orzo, and cook until golden, for 2 minutes.

2. Stir in garlic, courgettes, and carrot and cook for another 2 minutes.

3. Pour in the broth and mix in the zest of lemon. Take to simmer. Reduce heat to low levels and simmer for 10 minutes, or until liquid is absorbed and tender orzo is present.

4. Season with thyme and top with parmesan and serve.

Each Serving Provides:

Calories: 123 Total fat: 5 g saturated fat: 1.5 g monounsaturated fat: 3 g polyunsaturated fat: 0.5 g Cholesterol: 5 mg Sodium: 561 mg potassium: 97 mg Carbohydrates: 14 g Sugar: 1 g total fiber: 1.2 g total protein: 5.5 g Iron: 0.5 mg magnesium: 13 mg calcium: 95 mg vitamin a: 528 IU vitamin c: 3 mg vitamin d: 0 µg nutrition:

Almond-Crusted Tilapia

Yield: 8 servings

Ingredients

2 eggs 1 tsp of lemon pepper 1 tsp of garlic pepper 1 cup of almonds, ground 1 cup of freshly rubbed parmesan cheese 8 (6-ounce) tilapia fillets 1/4 cup of all-purpose dusting parmesan cheese eight sprigs of parsley eight lemon wedges

Recipe:

1. Beat the eggs until blended with the lemon pepper and the garlic pepper; set aside. Stir ground almonds together in a shallow dish with 1 cup of parmesan cheese until combined; set aside. Staub the flour from the tilapia fillets, and shake off the waste. Dip the tilapia into the egg, then press the mixture into the almond.

2. Cook tilapia in cooking spray in a large skillet over medium-high heat until golden brown on both sides, 2 to 3 minutes per hand.

Restrain heat to average. Sprinkle the tilapia with the remaining 1/2 cup of parmesan cheese, cover and continue to cook for about 5 minutes until the parmesan cheese has melted.

3. Move the tilapia to a serving bowl, and garnish with sprigs of parsley and wedges of lemon to eat.

Every Serving Provides:

Calories: 280 Total fat: 12 g saturated fat: 3,5 g monounsaturated fat: 6 g polyunsaturated fat: 2,5 g Cholesterol: 137 mg Sodium: 365 mg potassium: 512 mg carbohydrate: 7 g Sugar: 0 g total fiber: 1,5 g Protein: 36 g vitamin c: 4 mg vitamin d: 2 µg magnesium: 108 mg iron

Cauliflower Tacos with Chicken

Servings: 8

Ingredients

3 tablespoons of grapeseed oil or 3⁄4 teaspoons of chili powder 3⁄4 t of avocado oil

Instructions

1. Coat a large rimmed baking sheet with a cooking spray on it.
2. In a big bowl, mix butter, chili powder, cumin, onion powder, and 1/8 teaspoon salt. Remove the cauliflower and swirl top cover gently. Spread the cauliflower over the prepared pan in a single layer. Bake until tender and continue to brown for 15 to 20 minutes.
3. In the meantime, mix tomatoes, avocados, cilantro, jalapeños, onion, and the remaining 1/8 teaspoon salt in a small cup.
4. Top up the cauliflower with rice, chicken, and cheese. Bake for almost about 5 minutes until the cheese is melted.
5. Eat the cauliflower in tortillas with salsa and cabbage.

Health Details Serving Size

2 tacos per serving: 348 calories; 15.4 g total fat; 3.5 g saturated fat; 40 mg of cholesterol; 264 mg of sodium. 708 mg potassium; 35 g carbohydrate; 8.6 g fiber; 4 g sugar; 20.5 g protein; 438 iu vitamin A IU; 61 mg vitamin c; 94 mcg folate; 156 mg calcium; 2 mg iron; 75 mg magnesium

6.9 Marinades, Seasonings, and Rubs

Dry spices such as cayenne pepper flakes, thyme, cumin, nutmeg, all-spice and rubbed sage are perfect for making marinades and rubs for fish, poultry, lamb, pork and beef, as you can see in the following recipes.

The marinades and rubs in this segment allow the guesswork out of cooking with a taste. You can go for these recipes, or you can play with jazz

Condiments:

- Honey mustard, dijonnaise mustard, low-carb ketchup, light mayonnaise, jam, jelly, or honey. Consider low-sugar combinations if you have diabetes.
- Salsa made from fresh produce.
- Use Splenda sweetener or stevia instead of sugar, particularly if you have diabetes.
- Fresh lemon juice or lime juice.
- Store-brand cooking sprays made with olive oil and other unsaturated fat oils.
- Vinegar: balsamic, apple cider, sherry, champagne, white and red wine, and tarragon.
- Prepared horseradish.
- If you use soya sauce, chipotle sauce, or Worcestershire sauce, use only low-sodium versions or use it sparingly.
- Nice pickle relish.

Fresh herbs such as oregano, basil, rosemary, tarragon, and Italian flat-leaf parsley are now available in a variety of grocery stores. Cut fresh herbs for between $2.99 and $4.00, depending on where you shop. Tiny whole plants sell for around the same price or less and have continuous supply if they are watered and fed in a sunny kitchen window or a patio tub.

Island-Style Grilling Marinade

Yield: 24 servings

Ingredients

6 cloves garlic, coarsely minced 1/2 cup thin yellow onion 1 cup freshly squeezed orange juice 1/2 cup freshly squeezed lime juice 1/2 tsp ground cumin* 1 tsp dried oregano flakes* 1/2 tsp lemon pepper seasoning 1/2 tsp of newly ground black pepper* 1 tsp kosher salt 1/4 cup minced cilantro 1 tsp hot pepper sauce.

Recipe:

1. In a blender, pulse the garlic and onion until very thinly chopped. Add orange juice and lime juice; cumin, oregano, lemon pepper, black pepper, salt, cilantro, and hot pepper sauce to taste. Mix once well incorporated. Pour in the olive oil, then blend until smooth.

Note: beef and chicken should be marinated overnight, and the fish should only marinate for 1 hour.

Serve size: 2 tbsp

Per Serving Provides:

Calories: 86 total fat: 8.5 g saturated fat: 1.2 g monounsaturated fat: 6.5 g polyunsaturated fat: 0.8 g cholesterol: 0 mg sodium: 50 mg potassium: 103 mg carbohydrates: 2 g sugar: 0 g total fiber: 0.2 g iron: < 1 mg calcium: 5 mg iu vitamin c: 7 mg vitamin d:0 µg vitamin a: 3.9 iu magnesium: 2.5 mg nutrients

Fabulous Fajita Marinade

Yield: 8 servings

Ingredients

1/4 cup beer 1/3 cup fresh lime juice 1 tbsp olive oil two cloves garlic, 1 tbsp brown sugar 1 tbsp Worcestershire sauce 1 tbsp chopped cilantro 1/2 tsp ground cumin* salt, to taste

Recipe:

1. Stir milk, lime juice, olive oil, garlic, brown sugar, Worcestershire sauce, cilantro, cumin, and salt together to make the marinade; blend well.

2. Pour into a resealable plastic bag for use with marinade, attach up to 11/2 pounds of chicken breast and blend until the chicken is well coated.

Marinate in the fridge for at least 1 to 3 hours.

Serve size: 2 tbsp

Each Serving Provides:

Calories: 30 Total fat: 1.5 g saturated fat: 0.2 g monounsaturated fat: 1.2 g polyunsaturated fat: 0.1 g Cholesterol: 0 mg Sodium: 58 mg potassium: 26 mg carbohydrate: 3 g Sugar: 0 g dietary fiber: 0 g protein: < 1 g iron: < 1 mg calcium: 4.5 mg vitamin a: 0.5 IU vitamin c: 3.2 mg vitamin d:0 µg magnesium: 3 mg nutrients

Cajun Spice Rub

Yield: 4 servings

Ingredients

2 tbsp of paprika* 1 tbsp of cumin, ground* 1 tbsp of dried thyme four cloves of garlic, minced one onion, diced 1 tbsp of dried oregano* 1 tsp of black pepper* 1 tsp of cayenne pepper

Recipe:

1. Blend all the ingredients and rub them thoroughly on the skin. Enable meat to marinate for a minimum of 2 hours before cooking.

Each Serving Provides:

Calories: 45 Total fat: 0.75 g monounsaturated fat: < 1 g polyunsaturated fat: 0.5 g Cholesterol: 0 mg Sodium: 3.5 mg potassium: 228 mg saturated fat: < 1 g carbohydrates: 8 g carbohydrates: < 1 g total fiber: 2.5 g Iron: 2 mg vitamin c: 7.5 mg vitamin d:0 µg protein: 1.5 g magnesium: 20 mg calcium: 64 mg vitamin a: 245 iu nutrition

Honey Soy Sauce Salmon

Ingredients

12 oz skinless salmon one tablespoon olive oil for honey soy marinade four cloves garlic, minced two teaspoons ginger, diced 1/2 teaspoon red pepper one tablespoon olive oil

Instructions

1. Place all the marinade ingredients in a small bowl and combine thoroughly.
2. Add part of the marinade to the salmon. Save the other half of it for later.
3. Let the salmon marinate in the fridge for at least 30 minutes.
4. Heat oil in a medium oven. Apply salmon to the pan, but discard the marinade used. Cook salmon on one side for around 2-3 minutes, then turn over and cook for another 1-2 minutes.
5. Take salmon out of the oven. Add the remaining marinade to the frying pan and reduce to a thick sauce.
6. Serve the salmon with the sauce and the side of your favorite vegetables

Cilantro Lime Salmon

Servings 2 people Prep time 10 minutes Cook time 15 minutes total time 25 minutes calories 457 kcal

Ingredients

2 tablespoons olive oil two cloves garlic, 1 1/4 tablespoons lime juice 1/2 teaspoon salt or more to taste three filets cayenne pepper 1 lb salmon fillet two tablespoons chopped cilantro lime for garnishing

Directions

1. Preheat to 375f in the oven.

2. In a small cup, add olive oil, garlic, lime juice, salt, cayenne pepper, and half of the cilantro. Remove to blend correctly. Marinate the salmon with the mixture when the oven is preheating.

3. As soon as the oven is preheated, move the salmon to a baking sheet lined with aluminum foil or parchment paper and cook for about 15 minutes.

4. Extract the remaining chopped cilantro from the oven and garnish with the lime. Serve right away.

Nutrition Facts

Amount per serving (2 people) calories 457 calories of fat 252 percent daily value* fat 28g43 percent saturated fat 4g25 percent cholesterol 124 mg 41 percent sodium 682 mg 30 percent potassium 1141mg33 percent carbohydrates 2g1 percent protein 45g90 percent vitamin a 740iu15 percent vitamin c 4.9mg6 percent calcium 33mg3 percent iron 1.9 mg11 percent* per serving

6.10 Desserts

Brandy Apple Crisp

Yield: 6 servings

Ingredients

4 cups tart apples, peeled and diced 3 tbsp sugar 3 tbsp brandy 2 tsp lemon juice 1/2 tsp cinnamon 1/8 tsp nutmeg 3/4 cup dried oats 1/4 cup brown sugar 2 tbsp flour 2 tbsp margarine

Recipe:

1. In an 8-inch square-shaped baking pan, mix the first six ingredients. Toss well; put away.

2. In a small cup, add the oats, brown sugar, and flour. Cut in margarine until blended well. Sprinkle the mixture over the apples.

3. Bake for 45 minutes, at 350 ° f.

Serve size: 1/2 cup

Each Serving Provides:

Calories: 184 Total fat: 2 g saturated fat: 0.5 g monounsaturated fat: 0.5 g polyunsaturated fat: 1 g Cholesterol: 0 mg Sodium: 28 mg potassium: 202 mg carbohydrate: 40 g Sugar: 15 g dietary fiber: 4 g vitamin d:0 µg protein: 1.3 g Iron: 0.8 mg calcium: 22 mg vitamin a: 24 IU vitamin c: 8.8 mg nutrients

Green Tea Cakes

Note: the tea called for here is matcha, a powdered green tea used in the Japanese tea ceremony. Buying the highest-grade tea for this recipe is superfluous.

Yield: 12 servings

Ingredients

4 eggs one egg yolk, 1/2 cup of sugar 1/3 cup of cake flour 2 tbsp of cornstarch 2 tbsp of green tea 1/8 tsp of tartar 2 tbsp of sugar 6 tbsp of almond paste 1 cup of heavy cream four tsp of superfine sugar

Recipe:

1. Preheat oven to 450 degrees f.

2. Beat two whole eggs, three egg yolks, and seven spoonsful of sugar together with an electric mixer until thick and tripled in length, around 5 minutes.

3. Sift rice, cornstarch, and one spoonful of green tea together. Sift the mixture and fold in on broken eggs. Beat the egg whites with tartar cream until they form soft peaks. Beat until stiff, in the remaining one tablespoon of sugar. Bring the batter in. Spread mixture in a shallow 11-by-7-inch pan that has been grained and lined with wax paper that is greased and floured.

4. Bake to touch until lightly brown and springy. Cake edges loosen. Sprinkle with the sugar from the cookies, then cover with a kitchen towel and invert to a flat surface. Let's let it cool. Cut out 24 pieces of cake using a biscuit cutter or some other decorative cutter.

5. Paste the knead almond with one teaspoon green tea. Thinly spread out between sheets of plastic wrap. Print out 12 decorative forms using a small cookie cutter.

6. Slowly whisk heavy cream into superfine sugar and two teaspoons of green tea remaining, then beat until solid. To assemble cakes, sandwich two layers of cake with cream whipped around 1/4-inch green tea. Frost top and whipped cream sides, and cutouts of almond paste decorate. Chill to serve.

Edited and reproduced, with gourmania permission.

Serve size: 1 small four

Each Serving Provides

Calories: 197 Total fat: 12.5 g saturated fat: 5.5 g monounsaturated fat: 5.5 g polyunsaturated fat: 1.5 g Cholesterol: 98 mg Sodium: 30 mg potassium: 100 mg carbohydrate: 17 g Sugar: 6 g dietary fiber: 0.5 g Iron: 0.5 mg calcium: 43 mg vitamin a: 115 IU vitamin c: < 1 mg magnesium: 28 mg Protein: 4 g vitamin d: 0.5 g

Maple Crisp Bars

12 servings

Ingredients

1/3 cup of margarine 1 cup sugar 1 tsp maple extract 1/2 cup maple pancake syrup (not pure maple syrup) 8 cups puffed rice cereal

Recipe:

1. Melt the margarine in a large saucepan over medium heat. Add sugar, extract, and syrup and bring to a boil. Take off fire.

2. Incorporate rice, coat the sugar mixture thoroughly.

3. Push into a 13-by-9-inch greased baking pan. Slice into 20 bars.

Each Serving Provides:

Calories: 156 Total fat: 2 g monounsaturated fat: 0,5 g polyunsaturated fat: 1 g saturated fat: 0,5 g Cholesterol: 0 mg Sodium: 33 mg potassium: 40 mg carbohydrate: 34 g sugar: total fiber: < 1 g protein: 0,5 g Iron: 0,5 mg magnesium: 4,5 mg calcium: 10 mg vitamin c: 0 mg sugar: 10 g vitamin d: 0 µg magnesium:0,5 mg calcium: 10 mg vitamin a:22,5 iu.

Almond and apricot biscotti

Dietitian's tip: this double-baked cookie is a favorite with coffee or tea. Both wheat and nuts have mineral manganese and the antioxidant selenium.

Serves 24

Low Sodium

Low Fat

Ingredients

3/4 cup whole-3/4 cup all-1/4 cup brown sugar one teaspoon baking powder two eggs, lightly beaten two tablespoons 1 percent low-2 tablespoons canola oil two tablespoons dark honey 1/2 teaspoon almond extract 2/3 cup dried apricot extract

Instructions

1. Mix the flours, brown sugar, and baking powder in a big bowl. Just whisk to blend. Connect the eggs, milk, canola oil, honey, and the extract of the almonds. Stir it with a wooden spoon till the dough starts to come together. Attach the chopped almonds and apricots. Mix with floured hands until the mixture is well blended.
2. Place the dough on a sheet of plastic wrap and form by hand in a flattened log 12 inches long, 3 inches wide, and around 1 inch thick. Lift the plastic wrap on a nonstick baking sheet to invert the dough. Bake until lightly browned for 25 to 30 minutes. Switch to another baking sheet and cool for 10 minutes. Set the oven at 350 F.
3. Place the cooled log on the cutting board. Cut the diagonal crosswise into 24 slices half-inch long with a serrated knife. Put the slices on the baking sheet, cut the side down. Return to the oven and cook it until crisp, 15 to 20 minutes. Switch to the wire rack and let it cool down completely. Place it in an airtight jar.

Nutritional information per serving

Serving size: 1 cookie Calories 75 Total fat 2 g Saturated fat Trace Trans-fat Trace Unsaturated fat 1 g Cholesterol 15 mg Sodium 17 mg Total carbohydrate 12 g Dietary fiber 1 g Total sugars 6 g Added sugars 2 g Protein 2 g

Crane-fruit coffeecake with crumb topping

Dietitian tip: crumb topping is made with pecans, which are a good source of magnesium, potassium, zinc, copper, and phosphorus.

Amount of servings

Serves 10

Ingredients For topping:

1/4 cup whole-wheat flour 1/2 cup brown sugar 1/4 cup sliced pecans two teaspoons trans-free margarine, melted for the cake: 3/4 cup all-purpose flour 3/4 cup whole-wheat flour 3/4 cup sugar 1/2 teaspoon 1/4 teaspoon baking soda 1 1/4 teaspoon vanilla 8 oz. fat-free sour cream 2 oz.

Instructions

1. Cover a 10-inch round pan lightly with a cooking spray.
2. Within a small bowl, mix flour, brown sugar, and chopped pecans to make the topping. Pour into the melted margarine. Mix well — it's meant to look crumbling. Place it aside.
3. For a big bowl, mix flour, sugar, baking powder, and soda. Just whisk to blend.
4. For a separate cup, mix milk, sour cream, egg whites, and margarine. Use an electric mixer at low to medium speed, beat for around 2 minutes until well blended. Add flour mixture to a mixture of sour cream. Use a spoon, mix gently until smooth.
5. Place half of the batter in the oven. Top with some of the chopped fruit. Spread the remaining mixture on the berries. Sprinkle with the edges. Bake it until the wooden toothpick inserted into the middle comes out clean for about 45 minutes.
6. Cut the coffeecake into ten cubits and serve moist.

Nutritional overview per serving

Serving size: 1 slice Total fat 9 g Calories 281 Protein 4 g Cholesterol Trace Total carbohydrate 50 g Dietary fiber 3 g Unsaturated fat 4 g Saturated fat 1 g Trans-fat 0 g Sodium 198 mg Added sugars 25 g Total sugars 31 g

Fruity rice pudding

Dietitian's tip: prepare this fruity rice pudding ahead of time, refrigerate and eat cold. Or serve a warm dessert right from the oven.

Serves 8

Carb Low Fat

Ingredients

Two cups water 1 cup long-brown rice 4 cups evaporated fat-1/2 cup brown sugar 1/2 teaspoon lemon zest one teaspoon vanilla extract six egg whites 1/4 cup crushed pineapple 1/4 cup raisins 1/4 cup dried apricots, chopped

Directions

1. In a medium saucepan, bring 2 cups of water to a boil. Attach the rice and cook for about 10 minutes. Pour in a colander and rinse thoroughly.
2. Attach the evaporated milk and brown sugar to the same saucepan. Cook until it's soft. Connect the sugar, lemon zest, and vanilla extract. Simmer over low heat until the mixture is thick and the rice is tender for about 30 minutes. Remove from the heat and cool down.
3. In a small cup, whisk the egg whites together. Pour in the mixture of beans. Add pineapple, raisins, and legumes. Stir until blended well.
4. Power the oven to 325 ft. Cover a baking dish lightly with a cooking mist. Put the pudding and fruit mixture into the baking dish. Bake for about 20 minutes until the pudding is set. Serve hot or cold.

Nutritional analysis per serving

Serving size: around 1/2 cup Calories 257 Total fat 1 g Saturated fat <0.5 g Trans-fat 0 g Unsaturated fat <0.5 g Cholesterol 5 mg Sodium 193 mg Total carbohydrate 48 g Dietary fiber 1 g Added sugars 9 g Protein 17 g

7. Apples with dip

Dietitian tip: use fat-free instead of full-fat cream cheese, eliminate about 50 calories and 4 grams of mostly saturated fat

Serves 8

Low Fat

Healthy Carb

Ingredients

Eight ounces of fat-free cream cheese two tablespoons of brown sugar 1 1/2 teaspoons of vanilla two tablespoons of unsalted peanuts four medium or eight small apples, cored and sliced 1/2 cup orange juice

Instructions

1. Remove the cream cheese from the refrigerator to enable it to soften for around 5 minutes.
2. Mix brown sugar, vanilla, and cream cheese in a small cup. Mix until it's smooth. In the chopped peanuts, whisk.
3. Placed the sliced apples in another bowl. Drizzle the orange juice over the apples to prevent browning. Drain the apples and serve with the sauce.

Nutritional analysis per serving

Serving size: 1/2 medium apple and two tablespoons dip Total carbohydrate 19 g Dietary fiber 2.5 g Sodium 202 mg Saturated fat 0.5 g Trans-fat 0 g Healthy fat 2 g Cholesterol 3 mg Protein 6 g Unsaturated fat 1 g Calories 118 Added sugars 3 g Natural sugars 15 g.

Fruit and nut bar

Dietitian's tip: If you need a treat, try this safe indulgence.

Serves 24

Low Fat

Healthy Carb

Low Sodium

Ingredients

1/2 cup quinoa flour 1/2 cup oats 1/4 cup flaxseed flour 1/4 cup wheat germ 1/4 cup chopped almonds 1/4 cup chopped dried apricots (about five apricot halves) 1/4 cup chopped dried figs (about 5 figs) 1/4 cup honey 1/4 cup chopped dried pineapple two tablespoons cornstarch

Instructions

1. Mix all the ingredients, blend well. Push mixture to a half-inch thick pan. Bake for 20 minutes at 300 F. Cool and cut into 24 bits.

Nutritional analysis per serving

Serving size: 1 bar Total carbohydrate 11 g Dietary fiber 2 g Sodium 4 mg Saturated fat Trace Total fat 2 g Trans-fat 0 g Cholesterol 0 mg Protein 2 g Unsaturated fat 0.5 g Calories 70 Added sugars 3 g Total sugars 6

Banana & Peanut Butter Ice Cream

Per Serving Provides

Four serving

Ingredients

Four ripe bananas, sliced into 3 cm parts, then frozen 2 tbsp of almond milk 1 tbsp of organic peanut butter 1 tbsp of ground cinnamon 1 tbsp of dark chocolate, grated 1 tbsp of flaked almonds

Method

1. Tip the frozen bananas and almond milk in a blender. Mix to create a smooth consistency. Remove the peanut butter and cinnamon, then blend again. If you like, try and add more cinnamon.
2. Switch to a freezer-proof container and freeze for 1 hour. Remove from the freezer and serve with grated chocolate and flaked almonds.

Nutrition Facts:

Per serving kcal 169 fat 6g saturated 2 g carbohydrates 24 g sugars 22 g fiber 2 g protein 3 g salt 0 g

Savory spinach and feta oatmeal bowl

servings: 1

Ingredients

1/2 cup rolled oats 1 cup low-sodium chicken or vegetable broth olive oil two cloves garlic, minced 1 cup baby spinach one large egg one tablespoon feta cheese crumbs freshly ground black pepper, to taste per attach the oats and turn the heat down.

Instructions

1. Cook, stirring regularly until the oats, about 5 minutes, has absorbed all the liquid.

In the meantime, sauté the garlic and spinach in a small nonstick skillet. Remove the pan and set aside.

2. Spray the saucepan with the olive oil and cook the egg to the perfect doneness.
3. Place the oatmeal in a mug. Stir in spinach and feta. Top with a fried egg and a big crack of black pepper. Enjoy it!

Nutrition Facts Per Serving

309 calories 11 g fat 34 g carbohydrate 19 g

Chocolate Covered Banana-Walnut Bites

Servings: 8 (3 bits each)

Ingredients

2 medium bananas 4 ounces semi-sweet chocolate baking 1 1/2 tablespoon coconut oil 24 walnut halves

Preparation

1. Line a baking tray or cutting board with waxed paper. If possible, cover the waxed paper with a piece of tape.
2. Peel and slice the bananas into 1/2-inch slices.
3. Split the chocolate in half. Place the coconut oil and the microwave in a microwave-safe bowl for 30 seconds. Stir and repeat at intervals of 15 seconds until the chocolate is fully melted and smooth.
4. Working quickly, place the bananas on the tines of the fork and put them in the melted chocolate. I was using a spoon to pour chocolate over the rim until it has been thoroughly coated. Scrape the bottom of the fork over the side of the bowl to extract extra chocolate and use another fork to slip the banana slice over the prepared tray. Slowly press half of the walnut into the chocolate on top of the banana slice. If chocolate begins to get too thick, reheat as needed.
5. Chill the chocolate-covered bananas until the chocolate hardens for at least one hour. Serve it chilled. Every chocolate that is not eaten within 24 hours should be frozen for preservation in an airtight container.

Variations and Substitutions

Please read the label carefully when shopping for chocolate. This recipe has been created for semi-sweet chocolate baking. While certain varieties of semi-sweet chocolate chips can be substituted (those without milk in the list of ingredients), certain forms of baking chocolate, such as bittersweet, cannot be replaced.

Top some of the walnut bananas before diving, to change the appearance of the candies.

Pecan halves can be used instead of walnut halves.

Several other nuts or fruits can be dipped using the same technique; try dipping fresh strawberries, pineapples, or peanuts.

Cooking and Serving Tips

You may be able to immerse bananas in melted chocolate at first. So, as the amount of chocolate available reduces, you're going to have to tip the bottle and spoon up chocolate to spill over and cover the banana bits.

Nutrition Highlights (Per Serving)

141 calories 9 g fat 17 g carbs 2 g protein

Dark Chocolate Dipping Coconut Macaroons

Servings: 15 (1 cookie each)

Ingredients

2 large egg whites 1/4 cup granulated sugar 1/2 teaspoon vanilla extract 2 cups shredded coconut 1/4 cup dark chocolate chips

Preparation

1. Heat oven to 350f. Cover the baking sheet with parchment or a baking mat of silicone.
2. Whisk egg whites, sugar, and vanilla until foamy. Stir the coconut.
3. Scoop the mixture into1-inch balls and put it on a lined cookie sheet.
4. Bake for 15 minutes or until the macaroons are lightly golden. Clear from the oven and let it cool down.
5. In a small microwave-safe bowl, melt all the chocolate chips in a microwave at intervals of 30 seconds, stirring well until smooth.

6. Dip the bottoms of the macaroons in the melted chocolate and put on the parchment or silicone baking mat to dry until the chocolate has hardened.

Ingredient Variations and Substitutions

Use sliced dark chocolate instead of chocolate chips for a more indulgent taste.

Consider swapping the vanilla extract with the almond extract for the difference in taste.

Cooking and serving tips watch macaroons jointly at the end of cooking so that they do not burn.

Nutrition Highlights (Per Serving)

86 calories 4 g fat 12 g carbs 1 g protein

Strawberry-Rosemary Yogurt Pops

Ingredients

1 cup of chopped fresh strawberries two tablespoons balsamic vinegar two tablespoons strawberry preserves two fresh rosemary sprigs 1-1/2 cups vanilla yogurt six frozen pop molds or paper cups (3 ounces each) and wooden pop or lollipop sticks

Instructions

1. In a small bowl, mix strawberries, vinegar, preserves, and rosemary let stand for 30 minutes; discard the rosemary.
2. Spoon 2 tablespoons of yogurt and one tablespoon of the strawberry mixture into each mold or paper cup. Repeat layers, please. Top shapes and holders. Cover with foil and insert sticks through the foil while using containers. Freeze up to the company.

Health Facts

1 pop: 81 calories, 1 g fat (0 saturated fat), 3 mg cholesterol, 42 mg sodium, 16 g carbohydrate (15 g sugar, 1 g fiber), 3 g protein. Diabetic exchange: 1 starch.

Conclusion

None of the steps in this book are beyond the capacity of any human. Each phase is simple enough that there is no excuse for a person with high blood pressure not to recognize it and make it part of their everyday routine.

Proper diet and lifestyle are the main ways to combat cardiovascular disease. It's not that hard as much as you would imagine. Know, the increasing trend of your decisions is what counts. Make these necessary measures a part of your life to support your health and your heart in the long term. Keeping your diet in check — counting carbohydrates, reducing sugar, eating less salt — is essential. By following these simple tips and recipes, you can still eat well and control your conditions.

As there is no "magic bullet" to avoid high blood pressure, but a proper diet and daily exercise will go a long way to maintaining the blood pressure at a safe level. Here are our favorite high-blood-pressure-diet recipes for — you're not going to miss the salt! You may be consuming a lot of food, but your body may not be receiving the nutrients it requires to stay balanced. Nutrient-rich diets have minerals, proteins, whole grains, and other nutrients that are lower in calories. They can help you regulate your body weight, cholesterol, and blood pressure. In this cookbook, we discussed some delicious recipes that help you lower your blood pressure.

Dividends obtained by pursuing such measures would gradually make their way through every area of existence, for you would have met and disenfranchised an insidious enemy by simple, daily acts.

References

- Complementary and Alternative Treatments for High Blood Pressure. WebMD. Retrieved from https://www.webmd.com/hypertension-high-blood-pressure/guide/hypertension-complementary-alternative-treatments.
- How high blood pressure can affect your body. Mayo Clinic. Retrieved from https://www.mayoclinic.org/diseases-conditions/high-blood-pressure/in-depth/high-blood-pressure/art-20045868.
- High blood pressure (hypertension) - Diagnosis and treatment - Mayo Clinic. Mayoclinic.org. Retrieved from https://www.mayoclinic.org/diseases-conditions/high-blood-pressure/diagnosis-treatment/drc-20373417.
- Understanding Blood Pressure Readings. www.heart.org. Retrieved from https://www.heart.org/en/health-topics/high-blood-pressure/understanding-blood-pressure-readings.
- High blood pressure: What is high, symptoms, causes, and more. Medicalnewstoday.com. Retrieved from https://www.medicalnewstoday.com/articles/159283.
- Weight Loss and Blood Pressure Control (Pro) | Hypertension. Ahajournals.org. Retrieved from https://www.ahajournals.org/doi/10.1161/HYPERTENSIONAHA.107.094011.
- Managing Weight to Control High Blood Pressure. www.heart.org. Retrieved from https://www.heart.org/en/health-topics/high-blood-pressure/changes-you-can-make-to-manage-high-blood-pressure/managing-weight-to-control-high-blood-pressure.
- How high blood pressure can affect your body. Mayo Clinic. Retrieved from

https://www.mayoclinic.org/diseases-conditions/high-blood-pressure/in-depth/high-blood-pressure/art-20045868.
- Healthy High-Blood Pressure Recipes. Eating Well. Retrieved from http://www.eatingwell.com/recipes/18055/health-condition/high-blood-pressure/.
- Hypertension: 5 Breakfast Recipes To Manage High Blood Pressure. NDTV Food. Retrieved from https://food.ndtv.com/food-drinks/hypertension-5-breakfast-recipes-you-can-try-1886834.
- 13 Foods That Lower Blood Pressure. Healthline. Retrieved from https://www.healthline.com/health/foods-good-for-high-blood-pressure.
- High Blood Pressure and the DASH Diet. WebMD. Retrieved from https://www.webmd.com/hypertension-high-blood-pressure/guide/dash-diet#1.
- How to Reduce Your Blood Pressure Without Medication. Craving Something Healthy... Retrieved from https://cravingsomethinghealthy.com/how-to-reduce-blood-pressure-without-medication/.
- Hypertension (High Blood Pressure) Charts, Symptoms, Diet, & Medication. MedicineNet. Retrieved from https://www.medicinenet.com/high_blood_pressure_hypertension/article.htm#what_alternative_therapies_help_lower_and_mangage_high_blood_pressure.
- What is blood pressure and how is it measured?. Ncbi.nlm.nih.gov. Retrieved from https://www.ncbi.nlm.nih.gov/books/NBK279251/.

Printed in Great Britain
by Amazon